HOSPICE:
PRACTICE, PITFALLS,
AND PROMISE

HOSPICE: PRACTICE, PITFALLS, AND PROMISE

by
STEPHEN R. CONNOR

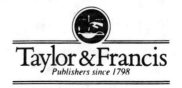
Taylor & Francis
Publishers since 1798

USA	Publishing Office:	Taylor & Francis 1101 Vermont Avenue, N.W., Suite 200 Washington, D.C. 20005-3521 Tel: (202) 289-2174 Fax: (202) 289-3665
	Distribution Center:	Taylor & Francis 1900 Frost Road, Suite 101 Bristol, PA 19007-1598 Tel: (215) 785-5800 Fax: (215) 785-5515
UK		Taylor & Francis Ltd. 1 Gunpowder Square London EC4A 3DE Tel: 171 583 0490 Fax: 171 583 0581

HOSPICE: Practice, Pitfalls, and Promise

1 2 3 4 5 6 7 8 9 0   E B E B   9 0 9 8 7

This book was set in Times Roman. The editors were Kelly Huegel and Kathleen Baker. Cover design by Michelle Fleitz.

A CIP catalog record for this book is available from the British Library.
∞ The paper in this publication meets the requirements of the ANSI Standard Z39.48-1984 (Permanence of Paper)

Library of Congress Cataloging-in-Publication Data

Connor, Stephen R.
   Hospice: practice, pitfalls, and promise / Stephen Connor.
      p.   cm.
   Includes bibliographical references.

   1. Hospice care.
I. Title
R726.8.C686   1997
362,1'756—dc21   96-28959
                                                                          CIP

ISBN 1-56032-512-7 (case)
ISBN 1-56032-513-5 (paper)

Dedication

This book is dedicated to all those who toil daily in caring for those of us at life's end.

Contents

Acknowledgments

This book would not have been possible without the support and encouragement of the sage Hannelore Wass, one of the Grand Dames of the death and dying movement. In many respects thanks is also due to the International Work Group on Death, Dying, and Bereavement, which has been a fertile ground for pushing the envelope of knowledge about the human encounter with death.

My family, Connie, Patrick, Eric, and Keara, have been incredibly patient in allowing me to hide in the basement over the past year to work at times they would rather have had my attention. I would also like to thank the following people who helped with their critical review or inspiration at points along the way: Dale Larson, Marcia Lattanzi-Licht, Connie Holden, Larry Beresford, Ira Byock, Neil and Marie Yates, Gary Bohannon, Chris Cody, Paul Gerard, Galen Miller, Inge Corless, Colin Murrey Parkes, Vickie Dornbusch, Doris Hartlage, Helen Donaldson, Gretchen Brown, Elaine Cox, Sarah Gorodezky, Phyllis Silverman, Jack Morgan and everyone in the International Work Group on Death, Dying, and Bereavement, Elaine Pirrone, Bernadette Capelle, and the great folks at Taylor and Francis.

Preface

This book describes the current practice of hospice care in the United States. In the past 25 years, the hospice movement has undergone major changes and has grown enormously. What was once a small rebellion against the way dying people were cared for has become a small health care industry. Hospices have improved the way people die. Still, the majority die in institutions, alone and in distress (SUPPORT Investigators, 1995).

There is a growing interest in the subject of care at the end of life. Society's aged population is growing larger than ever owing to postwar demographic trends and advances in medical treatment. People want to live as long as possible but expect life to be free from the indignities of advanced age. There must be quality of life in old age or a quick death. The current social debate on euthanasia is a reflection of the concern over how people die.

In spite of the impressive growth of hospice care, the great majority of people are not aware of the work hospices do. It is as if hospices are on the public's blind side. People do not seem to want to know what hospice does unless they need hospice services. Many professionals view hospice as a small effort that is too limited to have a large impact on how the majority of people die.

Whether hospices succeed in changing the way death is handled throughout society is still uncertain. Public policy currently limits reimbursement for hospice care in such a way that most of those who could benefit never get referred and more than half of those admitted are cared for for fewer than 30 days.

It will also be up to hospices themselves to go beyond their own limitations. If hospices prefer to remain comfortable with caring only for those patients who are easy to care for, the impact will be limited. Hospices must work harder at improving access for people of color and those with limited resources for caring.

After an initial period of growth following the creation of the Medicare Hospice Benefit in 1983, the number of hospices in the United States leveled off at about 2,000. In the past few years, there has been a renewed growth in both the number of hospices (2,900) and the numbers of people they serve (450,000).

There has also been considerable growth in European hospices since the fall of Soviet Communism (Saunders & Kastenbaum, 1997).

There is considerable need for those coming into the hospice movement and for those who are interested in end-of-life care to have an up-to-date grasp of where hospice care is today. This book is intended to give the reader an overall grasp of how hospice care is practiced, the challenges hospices currently face, and the direction the movement is taking.

This is the first book to give a full up-to-date account of how the hospice movement has developed in the United States. For those interested in how hospice care is organized and delivered, Part One, titled Practice, covers everything from history, to team functioning, to symptom management and psychospiritual care, to community education. The second part, Pitfalls, takes an honest and in-depth look at why the hospice movement has had limited success in changing the way most people die. The third part, Promise, points to how the movement can reach its potential to make dying in the United States not just something to endure but a time for life completion and growth.

In the first part, chapter 1 serves as an introduction. Hospice care is defined and a history of the movement is outlined. The 10 characteristics common to all hospices are described. The philosophical underpinnings of hospice care are discussed. An explanation of the needs of the whole patient is given in personal spheres, which include the physical, emotional, and spiritual needs of patients. An overview of the psychosocial issues facing dying patients is given. The standards that apply to hospice care are discussed. The chapter ends with a case that illustrates how effective hospice care can be.

In chapter 2, the role and work of each clinical team member are presented. The work of the administrative support team is also framed. This chapter explains how different types of team dynamics operate. Chapter 3 addresses pain and symptom management. Dying is universally associated with distress. Hospice makes it possible to face death by relieving these symptoms. Rather than discuss stages, it is helpful to examine the different trajectories the terminally ill patient faces. These trajectories may be associated with different disease types. Pain is the most feared symptom. How hospice manages pain and other common symptoms is presented. The concept of quality of life is discussed, along with the controversy about how it is measured. Successful hospice care depends on caregivers' involvement in care delivery. How hospice staff educate patients and families is described. This chapter ends with a case illustration of good symptom management in a difficult case.

Chapter 4 concerns psychosocial and spiritual issues. The various stage theories and their limitations are discussed. Death occurs on a number of dimensions. The loss of social identity, psychological adjustment to impending death, and spiritual issues faced by the dying are explored. Dying may involve certain psychological tasks, which are examined. The International Work Group on Death, Dying, and Bereavement has formulated assumptions and principles for psychosocial care of dying persons and their families. These principles are reviewed here. The concept of acceptance of death is evaluated and presented in a case example.

Chapter 5 is on grief and bereavement. One of hospice's unique services is to provide extensive bereavement support and counseling to families. The routine follow-up with hospice families is described as is that provided to the community at large. Special considerations for grieving children are given. Included is an examination of how pathological grief reactions can be distinguished from normal grief reactions and an update on current research into predicting poor outcomes. My study on hospice's impact on the use of health care resources by widowers is included. The chapter concludes with cases illustrating treatment of complicated grief.

Many hospices have extensive community education programs to increase awareness of the needs of dying patients and their families. In chapter 6, this little-discussed aspect of hospice care is highlighted. In spite of efforts by hospices, the public remains unaware of the issues faced by terminally ill persons. This is due, at least in part, to a practiced avoidance of terminal illness by the public. Hospice has found a receptive audience in school systems that are eager to help children learn about and respond to death in healthier ways. Hospice has a role in helping the community to respond to disasters and traumatic deaths. Debriefing and posttrauma response is discussed. The medical community is in continual need of education about the principles of palliative care. Finally, in this chapter the use of ''common concern'' support groups by hospice is discussed.

Chapter 7 begins the second part of the book and discusses the unique aspects of managing a hospice. It is a business, and it is a calling. The people who work in hospices are drawn there for a variety of reasons, some noble, some problematic. Running a hospice calls for more than just business skills. There is much emphasis on creating an organizational climate where staff and volunteers are supported and empowered. The role of volunteers in hospice care is explained. Standards of the National Hospice Organization are summarized, along with difficulties in hospice accreditation. The chapter ends with specific examples of problems seen in starting and running hospices.

Chapter 8 includes a brief history of how the U.S. health care system has dealt with dying patients, the development of the Hospice Medicare Benefit, and other forms of hospice coverage. Also discussed is the problem of determining prognosis in terminally ill people, including recent work on the development of clinical parameters for determining prognosis in nonmalignant terminal illness. Also examined is how entry into the mainstream of health care has resulted in certain problems of inflexibility for hospices and a tendency toward overestimation of hospice's ability to manage all aspects of the dying experience. The problem of measuring the quality of care given to dying patients is discussed, along with problems in conducting research in the hospice setting that has limited acceptance by the scientific community. This lack of acceptance extends to the physician community, which has viewed palliative care as unimportant and resists efforts to recognize it as a subspecialty. Recent efforts to reform the health care system and their impact on hospice are mentioned, along with a discussion of the impact of the development of for-profit hospices.

Chapter 10 examines the extensive impact of denial and avoidance on the ability of hospice to achieve its mission. Some historical perspectives on denial in American culture are given. The limitations of stage theories of denial are given, and my research into the effects of psychosocial intervention on denial is discussed. How to effectively work with hospice patients is illustrated through case examples.

In the final chapter of Part Two is an examination of hospice's position on euthanasia. Explored are the motivations for suicide requests and situations involving apparent unbearable suffering. How hospices and society have responded to these most difficult circumstances is presented. A discussion of efforts to legalize physician-assisted suicide and its impact on hospice is given. A case illustrating the above points is presented.

Chapter 11 begins the third part of the book, describing what is unique about hospice care. Hospice is a unique blend of services that aim to work in a truly collaborative fashion. The traditional hierarchical model with the physician as central figure is replaced by one in which the patient is central and all services have relative significance depending on patient need. Hospice, more than any other provider, seeks to empower patients and families to meet their goals. There is an emphasis on deinstitutionalization of care and prevention of distress rather than reaction to inevitable problems. Certainly, provision of spiritual care, in-depth psychosocial support, and bereavement care are unique aspects of hospice. The people who come to work in hospices tend to be dedicated in ways unlike other providers. There is a tendency to go beyond expectations and to see work as an expression of a higher self. Hospice's emphasis on quality of life goes beyond the notion of providing discipline-specific services. It is a community of people who are dedicated to helping each family find its way through life's most difficult transition.

Chapter 11 also includes a section on growth at the end of life and a summary of the work of Ira Byock, MD, on developmental landmarks and tasks for the end of life.

Chapter 12 looks at how hospice care is evaluated. In spite of the difficulties inherent in hospice research, there have been a number of important studies of hospice effectiveness that are reviewed. I discuss how hospices can evaluate themselves both internally and externally. Work on evaluating outcomes of hospice care is summarized. Finally, there is a look at quality improvement and clinical pathway development efforts in hospices.

The final chapter on the future of hospice care is an exploration of the nature of hospice care, whom its patients ought to be, and how it fits in the health care system. Questions addressed include the following: Should hospice strive to become obsolete or will there always be a need for a specialized care for the dying? Is hospice for terminally ill patients only or for all with life-threatening illnesses? Will physicians embrace palliative care as a respected science?

This book may be particularly useful to hospice programs that are growing and bringing in new staff and volunteers. This text gives detailed information that can greatly help orient new hospice caregivers, not only to the necessary knowledge of hospice practice but to many of the more subtle issues and aspects of hospice care that can take staff months or years to understand.

The text may also be useful to educators who are teaching about hospice care in an undergraduate or community college setting. There are sample questions and study activities to assist teachers in applying the text to coursework.

Hospice care is of growing importance to society as our culture struggles with how to provide compassionate end-of-life care to a growing segment of the population. Many different professionals can obtain an accurate understanding of hospice care through this book.

Throughout this book are case illustrations and stories that come from actual experiences in hospice. Names have been changed to preserve confidentiality.

Part One

Practice

In this section, the reader will learn the fundamentals of hospice care as it is currently practiced in the United States. Some information on hospice practices in Europe is included for contrast and comparison.

Chapter One

So What Is Hospice, Anyway?

DEFINITION

There is much confusion over the meaning of the word *hospice*. Some believe a hospice is a place where people die. Others simply associate the word with death and are uncomfortable. Those who have used hospice think of it as caregiving in the finest tradition: care that is both competent and compassionate—care provided to people facing death by people unafraid to face death.

In truth, hospice is all the above and much more. The word *hospice* comes from the Latin word *hospitium,* meaning hospitality, and from the old French word *hospes,* or host. Webster's defines hospice as a shelter or lodging for travelers, children, or the destitute, often maintained by a monastic order. Today, it is a word used to describe a program of care for individuals and their families facing a terminal illness. The National Hospice Organization (NHO, 1993) defines hospice as

a coordinated program providing palliative care to terminally ill patients and supportive services to patients, their families, and significant others 24 hours a day, seven days a week. Comprehensive/case managed services based on physical, social, spiritual, and emotional needs are provided during the last stages of illness, during the dying process, and during bereavement by a medically directed interdisciplinary team consisting of patients/families, health care professionals and volunteers. Professional management and continuity of care is maintained across multiple settings including homes, hospitals, long term care and residential settings. (NHO, 1993)

THE HOSPICE MOVEMENT

Why is there a hospice movement? Throughout the 20th century, modern medicine has transformed the experience of dying from a part of daily life to a highly technological event. Before the widespread use of antibiotics following the Second World War, people died at a younger age and with less forewarning. Physicians could do little but visit and attend to the dying by relieving their suffering. People were less apt to be rushed to the hospital, and they convalesced at home with the help of their families.

After the Second World War, great advances were made in the science of medicine. Many pharmaceutical agents were developed to treat illness, and techniques and equipment were invented to ward off the dying process. A seemingly unconscious goal was the elimination of death. Dying patients were not acknowledged. People died in institutions, not at home. They did not die, they "expired." They had to be kept alive at all costs; to do less was a failure.

Many health care professionals were frustrated in this climate. Many family members of the dying were angry at the way care was depersonalized. Physicians and nurses were not trained to care for the dying. Most were uncomfortable with the notion. They tended to visit dying patients less often. Unrealistic optimism lead to a "conspiracy of silence" where the patient and medical staff knew the truth but withheld it from that patient (Glaser & Strauss, 1965). There was a widespread belief that to tell a patient she or he was dying would cause harm and lead to premature demise. Patients were expected to follow physicians' recommendations without question. If death occurred, it was an unintended event.

In this atmosphere of denial, many caregivers were dissatisfied. There had to be a better way to treat the dying. The United States in the 1970s was a society undergoing rapid change. Most institutions were being challenged, and people were experimenting with new ways to solve old problems. Cancer patients were demanding more participation in treatment decisions, and support groups were being formed to give information and counseling. Those involved in treating dying patients began hearing about a new approach to care being used in the United Kingdom called hospice.

BRIEF HISTORY

It is generally held that the first hospices were established in the 11th century by the Crusaders. Until that time, incurable patients were not admitted to places of healing. Their presence was viewed as a detriment to the healing process of others. The first hospices were places where travelers to and from the Holy Land were cared for and refreshed. Travelers as well as the sick and the dying were cared for. The Knights Hospitallers of St. John of Jerusalem founded a way station in Jerusalem for sick and weary pilgrims but were forced by the Crusades to move on to Tyre, and then to Acre, and eventually to the island of Cyprus.

The Hospitallers were recognized by the Pope as a military order in 1113 and gained support carrying pilgrims to and from the Holy Land. In 1309, they stormed Rhodes and held it for two centuries. It was here that they founded a hospice hospital that cared for the sick, for travelers, and for incurables. The knights developed a special tradition of caring for our lords the sick and dying. They were treated royally with great dignity and the finest foods, linens, and treatments the order could offer. The knights themselves, having taken a vow of poverty, dined on plainer fare and were under strict orders forbidding any mistreatment. Their spiritual foundations were nourished by their work tending to the sick and dying.

The hospice tradition of the Middle Ages passed into history. It was reborn in the 17th century through the efforts of St. Vincent de Paul, who founded the Sisters of Charity in Paris. They opened a number of houses to care for orphans, the poor, the sick, and the dying. The Irish Sisters of Charity founded Our Lady's Hospice for care of the dying in Dublin. In 1900, the Irish Sisters founded a convent in London's East End. Their ministry included visiting the sick in their homes. In 1902, they founded St. Joseph's Hospice for the dying poor. More than 50 years later, Cicely Saunders came to work there and developed her approaches to managing pain and the total needs of dying patients. Her philosophy of using a team to treat the whole person has become the foundation for hospice care throughout the world.

Dame Saunders, who trained first as a nurse, then as a social worker, and finally as a physician, envisioned a center for excellence in care of the dying patient. This center included teaching and research facilities. In 1967, she opened St. Christopher's Hospice outside London in Sydenham. As matriarch of the worldwide hospice movement, she has inspired caregivers to carry on her mission of caring for the dying.

Hospice first came to North America in 1971. Hospice Inc., in New Haven, Connecticut, was founded, and a home care service began there in 1973. By 1980, Hospice Inc. had opened a 44-bed inpatient facility in Branford, Connecticut, exclusively for the care of dying patients. In the mid-1970s, a small but committed hospice movement had begun to take shape throughout the United States and Canada. From Marin, Monterey, and Fresno in California to Tucson, Arizona; to Boonton, New Jersey; to Montreal, Quebec, Canada; to St. Luke's Hospital in New York, various models of hospice care were being tested.

The National Hospice Organization was founded in 1978 and began holding annual educational conferences. The first national directory of hospices was published in 1978, with 1,200 hospices listed. The U.S. hospice movement had a slant distinctly toward home care. Most Americans surveyed showed a preference for dying in their homes. There was a greater emphasis on use of volunteers and more focus on psychological preparation for death than in English hospices.

In the early years of the American hospice movement, reimbursement for hospice care was limited to payment for components of care such as acute hospitalization and home health agency services. In 1982, hospice care was added as a Medicare benefit. This benefit eventually encouraged tremendous growth in the number of patients served by hospices and brought some standardization to the types of services a hospice could deliver.

The 1996–97 Guide to the Nation's Hospices (NHO, 1996a) includes more than 2,900 organizations providing hospice services. Today, approximately 40% of hospices are independent corporations, whereas 37% are divisions of a hospital and 21% are divisions of a home health agency. In 1992, 37% of all people who died of cancer in the United States were under the care of hospices. The number of noncancer terminal patients served by hospices was growing until recently. Data in 1992 reported 22% of hospice's patients had noncancer diagnoses. In 1995, the percentage had risen to 40%, though it is believed to be declining due to government scrutiny over determination of prognosis. Although people with AIDS have difficulty accepting the use of hospice, in 1992, 31% of those who died received hospice care.

The most recent in-depth census data on hospices from the NHO reveals that in 1996 there were 2,914 operating hospices. Of those responding to the census, 81% were licensed and 90% were Medicare certified. Another 6% had certification pending. Hospices who use only volunteers continue to operate and represent about 6% of programs (NHO, 1996c).

A total of 31% of programs were accreditated by the Joint Commission of Accreditation of Health Care Organizations (JCAHO), and 3% were accreditated by the Community Health Care Accreditation Program. Another 29% of programs planned to apply for accreditation by the end of 1997; 23% did not plan to.

A total of 87% of programs were nonprofit entities, and 10% were for profit. The remaining 3% were governmentally controlled. The vast majority of hospices are still small programs with an average daily patient census of 43, an average of 223 admissions a year, and an average revenue of $2,000,000. There is some skewing of the group, with some very large hospices. A more accurate number is the median revenue for a hospice, $615,000 per year, including $35,000 in charitable contributions. Median admissions per year are 108 people.

The greatest source of revenue for hospices is Medicare reimbursement, which accounts for 74% of income. Another 10% comes from Medicaid and 13% from private insurance payments (NHO, 1996c).

The length of time under hospice care appears to be declining. The average length of stay in 1995 in the census was 52 days. Here again there is skewing, with a small number of people with long stays in hospice. The median is a more accurate measure of central tendency in hospice length of stay and is only 29 days.

Hospices are beginning to merge and form partnerships. A total of 10% reported merging with or being purchased by another organization as of July 1, 1996. Another 25% indicated that chances of merger or purchase by another organization were certain, very likely, or somewhat likely in the next 24 months. A total of 43% have formed strategic partnerships with other organizations, mainly with home health agencies (45%) or other hospices (41%) (NHO, 1996c).

Hospices are seeking contracts with managed care. A full 62% have contracts with managed care, and 61% are currently negotiating agreements. Only 7% of programs have signed capitation agreements to provide services for covered lives. There is considerable interest in providing services outside of the current definition of 6-month prognosis. Thirty-one percent of programs are operating special-care or defined prehospice programs.

The vast majority of hospices reported that they are currently in compliance with NHO standards (95%), and 93% reported that they are active in their state hospice association; however, only 65% reported that they are active in the national association.

Many believe that hospices do not serve patients without primary caregivers. Hospices would serve more who lack caregivers if more resources were available; however, almost 6% of patients served in hospices in 1995 did not have a primary caregiver.

CHARACTERISTICS

In the United States, a set of characteristics has been developed that universally describes the essential components of a hospice program. Since the mid-1970s, these 10 characteristics have been a necessary part of every hospice.

1 *The patient and family are the unit of care.* Hospices do not admit a patient in isolation. They see each patient as part of a family system. Often the family's needs are equal to or greater than the dying person's. By family, I mean those bonded to the patient by blood or emotional ties, the patient's most immediate attachment network.

2 *Care is provided in the home and in inpatient facilities.* The philosophy of hospice care is to allow people to die where they want. Most people prefer to be cared for in their homes; others need or chose to be in a facility. Hospice care should be available to patients in all settings.

3 *Symptom management is the focus of treatment.* Hospice patients understand that there is no definitive cure for their illnesses. They seek relief from pain and other symptoms of terminal illness. Hospice care is directed at treating the symptoms, not curing the disease.

4 *Hospice treats the whole person.* A dying person is not just a physical entity. Hospice care is designed to address physical, social, psychological, spiritual, and practical needs of dying patients.

5 *Services are available 24 hours a day, 7 days a week.* People die and have problems at all hours of the day and night. Hospice services are available on weekends and at 2:00 a.m. if needed.

6 *Hospice care is interdisciplinary.* The hospice team draws on the skills of people in a variety of disciplines who work collaboratively in meeting the patients' various needs. The hospice team includes physicians, nurses, social workers, and other mental health professionals, chaplains, therapists, and volunteers.

7 *Hospice care is physician directed.* The patient's attending physician must determine that the patient has an incurable condition with a limited life expectancy and must order all palliative care delivered. The hospice medical director oversees the care of all hospice patients and supplements the services of the attending physician.

8 *Volunteers are an integral part of hospice care.* Dying persons respond uniquely to volunteers. Volunteers work with people facing death out of human concern. Often they have experienced death in their lives and can appreciate how hard it is for families to handle difficult situations.

9 *Services are provided without regard to ability to pay.* Hospices meet the needs of terminally ill people in their communities and do not deny services on the basis of inability to pay. When reimbursement is exhausted, care to the patient is not diminished.

10 *Bereavement services are provided to families on the basis of need.* Hospice provides a program of bereavement support to all families for at least a year following a patient's death. Grief counseling is begun before a patient's death. Bereavement support may also be extended to those grieving in the community at large.

Admission to a hospice program is generally limited to those diagnosed with a terminal illness with a limited life span. To become a hospice patient means that at some level patients acknowledge that they cannot be cured of their illnesses. This is not to say that one must abandon all hope to be served by hospice. Hospices view their role as one that accompanies another on life's last journey. No one knows how long any patient has to live; one can only help them to live until death comes.

PHILOSOPHY

Many of the underpinnings of hospice care can be found in the philosophy of humanism. Any individual has the right to determine how to be treated when facing a terminal illness. Those who refuse to acknowledge the possibility of their death usually do not want the services of a hospice. They choose to continue efforts to be cured through aggressive medical intervention. Hospice patients prefer to concentrate on living as comfortably as they can and keeping the troubling symptoms of illness at bay.

The right to determine treatment has many implications for hospice care. It means that the person may choose not to die in his or her own home, may express continued ambivalence about treatment and prolongation of life, and may change his or her mind along the way. This requires hospice workers to remain flexible with patients as they travel along this last journey. In a recent Gallop Poll (NHO, 1992), 9 out of 10 people said they preferred to be cared for and to die in their own homes, and 3 out of 4 were very interested in hospice care when it was described to them.

A philosophy of humanism requires hospice workers to accept patients unconditionally. As hospice grows and serves a larger segment of the population as a whole, a wider variety of life-styles are seen, including some families whose values conflict with hospice workers' or whose lifelong history of dysfunction is difficult to tolerate. Hospice workers learn not only to tolerate but to respect individual differences in the human family. Hospices still have a long way to go to fully understand different cultures and their responses to death. They will still continue to promote a reverence for the universal human experience of preparation for death.

This respectful reverence began with the Knights Hospitallers' admonitions about how to care for "our lords the sick and dying." It is a core part of hospice philosophy that to approach the human encounter with death is to face what is noblest in humanity. Even the poorest in spirit can be transformed by the experience.

One of the critical advantages to the hospice approach is that it allows an opportunity to prepare for death. If one only seeks a cure for the disease against all odds, the reality of impending death is never faced. Facing the imminent possibility of the end of life creates important opportunities. It allows people to say good-bye to the ones they love, it allows them to resolve any interpersonal conflicts that have been left incomplete, it allows a time for review of their lives to perhaps find meaning, and it allows practical preparations for death, including all the paperwork and bureaucracy of death that is so hard on survivors afterward.

Unlike those who would pit theology against humanism, hospice philosophy embraces the spiritual life. Hospices were founded by religious orders, and many who work in hospices see their work as an expression of their spiritual values; seeking to relieve suffering, to help others come closer to God while preparing for death, and to put service above self are hallmarks of the religious life.

PERSONAL SPHERES

Human beings are complex organisms who operate simultaneously on a number of levels. Maslow's (1967) conceptualization of the hierarchy of needs helps one to understand the dilemma of the dying patient. One's physical needs must be tended to before one can focus on emotional needs. Spiritual needs are difficult to attend to if emotional needs are unmet.

The hospice approach recognizes this paradigm of wholeness. It first focuses on the physical comfort of its patients. Control of their symptoms is paramount. A patient must have pain controlled, nausea and vomiting relieved, bowels functioning, mind alert, skin intact, and breathlessness relieved before anything else. Once there is a physical sense of well-being and the environment is safe, emotional reactions can emerge.

People have many and varied reactions to dying. Every human emotion can be evoked. The ability to express feelings is central to recovery from trauma. Most people also need a great deal of information about their illnesses. Those who are cognitively oriented best handle difficulty with facts and forewarnings. Thoughts and feelings need expression before questions of deeper meaning can be considered.

If comfort is achieved and thoughts and feelings are worked through, some have an opportunity to find meaning before death. Some find it in their religious beliefs, others in their philosophy of life. Life is examined and reviewed, and a sense of perspective is gained. Each person seeks to understand his or her personal reason for being. Those patients who have this awareness can use this time between living and dying to shed the distractions of daily life and find their meaning.

Hospice care means recognizing a person as a whole being, not just a body part. In medicine, it is not uncommon to hear patients referred to as "the lung patient" or "the liver patient." In hospice, each person is recognized as a unique being with a life history and perspective. It is recognized that illness affects not only the body but the soul and psyche as well.

PSYCHOSOCIAL ASPECTS OF HOSPICE CARE

One way of understanding how people react to the knowledge of impending death is to look at loss theory and how people grieve. A dying person must face many losses in the time leading up to physical death. These small deaths include the loss of being a healthy person, of being able to work, of friends, of being able to care for oneself, of a future self, and so forth. These losses vary depending on age and which losses have already occurred during the life span.

How the dying person reacts to these losses will vary widely depending on many factors. There is no predictable road map to the grieving process. Each human being faces death in his or her own way, some with complete avoidance, others with terror, and some with anticipation. All the reactions and stages that have been proposed in the literature are ways in which people react or cope, but these reactions and stages do not tell how one individual will respond. There is no such thing as a typical death.

When someone loses a loved one, they must react to a disequilibrium that occurs. One of the general schemas from loss theory (Bowlby, 1980/81) that helps us understand this is the progression from protest, to despair, to detachment, to resolution or integration. It is common for people to protest the reality of the loss in a variety of ways. When none of this protest changes anything, they may begin to despair; as they tire of despairing, they sometimes begin to detach themselves from the relationship. Gradually, people integrate the loss into who they are and go on with life.

The difficult issue for the dying person is that there is little time to go through this progression. With malignancy, there is usually a short period from the point at which there is no more treatment available to death. This is certainly less than 6 months and is more often weeks to a few months, sometimes only days. In some cases, attempts at curative treatment continue until the moment of death.

There are a number of important issues that need to be kept in mind by those who work with people facing death. The first is to always remember that the person dying has to set the agenda. Hospice workers cannot impose their ideas of how one should react or respond. They may have the idea that dying people should always say good-bye to their families. This is laudable, but in each life there are many different relationships, and not all of them can be resolved. All people die with some unfinished business.

Second, hospice workers should direct their efforts at tying up loose ends, not uncovering issues. If they are fortunate enough to be invited by the patient into a therapeutic relationship, they must realize that it is never therapeutic to open up issues that they will not be able to work through with the patient. Relationships with the dying have a unique quality. Because they know their time is limited, patients can more quickly develop a close working relationship. Transference can occur earlier and more intensely. Another way of seeing this is that people who are dying cut through superficiality and want to deal with important issues in their lives. It is tempting to go with them and to want to do in-depth psychotherapy. It is critical to be careful to work only toward resolution.

Third, it is helpful to understand that people who are dying are a reflection of society as a whole: Some are insightful, others are not; some are intelligent, others are not; some are caring, others may be insensitive or just plain mean. Hospice cares not just for normal folks but also for people who have a long history of mental illness or disability. It is helpful to bring clinical knowledge of how to respond to and treat emotional problems.

It is also very important not to pathologize the dying process. Death is not a mental illness. People facing terminal illness are under one of life's greatest stresses. They may use their less adaptive ways of coping under this stress. They may act out and be very difficult to be around. It is best to understand this and to not take it personally. Working with the dying demands great tolerance and patience.

STANDARDS

Hospices, in their early development, resisted the idea of standardization. The creation of the modern hospice has required as much creativity as it has scientific knowledge. To attempt to codify the operations of a hospice could have the unintended effect of preventing the hospice from responding to the most significant needs of dying patients and their families in a particular locale. The founders of the hospice movement tended to be leaders with tremendous personal integrity and moral character. Unselfish devotion to the needs of the dying was their primary motivation. There was not too much concern with needing to protect a vulnerable public.

As the hospice movement has grown, there are some who view hospice's reputation for excellent care and good works with envy. The word *hospice* conjures up the best qualities of the helping profession. Just using the word helps to raise funds. The proliferation of hospices in the United States and other countries has caused concerns about how to maintain some measure of quality. New programs are formed with the idea that any service to dying patients means hospice care. Older hospice programs sometimes cling to outmoded palliative care concepts and practices that deprive their patients of services and more effective symptom management.

It was inevitable that the practice of hospice care would need to be specified in operating standards that would help to say what hospice is and thus what it is not. A standard of practice is developed from a consensus among experts about how services need to be delivered for good outcomes to occur. There are principally four types of standards in health care.

Licensing standards generally specify the minimum requirements needed to deliver services to the public. They are concerned with safety and protection of the consumer. Certification requirements are standards that must be met to receive payment for services delivered. Professional association standards are developed to further raise the level of quality of services provided and are those deemed necessary to belong to a recognized national or regional organization that represents providers. Finally, accreditation standards are developed to reflect the state of the art in services provided and are voluntarily sought by organizations wishing to hold themselves out to the public as providers who meet the highest quality of care.

The characteristics of hospices previously mentioned were the first standards in that they all needed to be present for an organization to be considered a hospice. One of the first groups to develop guidelines for care of dying patients was the International Work Group on Death, Dying, and Bereavement. A set of *Assumptions and Principles Underlying Standards of Care for the Terminally Ill* were developed and finalized by this group in 1978.

This document and others were used by NHO to develop the first *Standards for a Hospice Program of Care*. These standards were revised and disseminated a number of times in the early 1980s and were published in 1987.

In 1984, JCAHO (1984) initiated an accreditation program for hospices. The standards for this program were developed with the hospice community under a grant from the Kellogg Foundation. For 6 years, the program accredited mostly hospital-based hospice programs. It was discontinued in 1990 by JCAHO because of cost and lack of participation by the larger hospice community.

In response to the discontinuation of JCAHO's program, NHO saw the need to develop more extensive standards for its members. NHO's Standards and Accreditation Committee was charged with rewriting the *Standards of a Hospice Program of Care*. These standards were published in 1993 and currently represent the best in hospice care.

Beginning in 1995, JCAHO decided to offer accreditation again to hospice programs. The new hospice accreditation program is a part of JCAHO's Home Care Accreditation Program (JCAHO, 1994). Some hospices are concerned that JCAHO's new program attempts make them look like home health agencies and does not include adequate detail in areas central to good hospice practice.

JCAHO's new hospice accreditation process follows the format established for all programs accredited by the joint commission. The 11 chapters developed through their "agenda for change" attempt to capture those areas of operation that are the most important processes for any health care provider. They address processes relating to care of the patient as well as operation of the organization. Although the standards may not be specific enough, it is important that hospices are able to meet the same standards that the rest of the health care system is addressing.

CASE ILLUSTRATION

Mary

The following case history illustrates a hospice scenario with a well-functioning family that was able to fully benefit from hospice intervention.

Mary was a 68-year-old patient with metastatic breast cancer who was referred to hospice by her physician while in the hospital for disease recurrence. She had failed chemotherapy and was having pain problems as a result of bone metastases. She lived with her spouse of 45 years, John, who was very supportive but had recently had a minor heart attack. They had two grown children who had families of their own but were in the area and were very supportive. The referring physician had given them the facts of her condition but sensed that they were having difficulty accepting her condition and prognosis.

During hospice intake, their hopes and fears about her condition were explored. Mary was very fearful about her spouse. She was afraid her condition might aggravate his heart condition. In their families of origin, each of their fathers had died before their mothers. They believed that it was abnormal for her to die before him. While exploring these issues, they were able to understand why they were having difficulty facing the reality of her condition. As we talked, more it became apparent that each knew the seriousness of her condition, but each was afraid to level with the other for fear that it would be harmful.

As this conspiracy of silence was dropped, their communication improved and they were able to make plans. Her pain was controlled by means of oral morphine and nonsteroidal anti-inflammatory medication. The relief of improved communication with her family also seemed to help lessen her pain. She came to understand that her husband was devoted to her and that his participation in caregiving would not worsen his health.

She remained stable for a few months and gradually began to weaken. During this time, the nurse visited regularly and taught her and the family what to expect as her condition worsened. The chaplain visited and helped her to explore a relationship with God that had grown distant in her later years. A home health aide was assigned to begin providing personal care. A volunteer visited weekly to become acquainted and to help with errands.

One evening 9 weeks after her admission, our on-call nurse received a call from Mary's husband that she was having pain. The nurse went to the house to assess and after talking with the physician on call increased her morphine; the next day, her regular nurse visited and found Mary to be comfortable but weaker. She was spending more time in bed now. The social worker asked for a family meeting with her children to talk about how to help care for Mary as she got sicker. A schedule was made out so John would have help in caring for her. A hospital bed was set up at home in the living room so she could be cared for in the common living area. Once a week, the volunteer agreed to be available to stay with Mary for 4 hours so John could go out during the day to shop.

As the next few weeks progressed, Mary gradually became weaker. Her children and grandchildren spent time with her, and she reminisced about their lives. Her discomfort increased but was controlled with adjustments in her medications. She began to sleep more and to talk less with her family. Her hospice nurse held a family meeting to describe again how the dying process normally progressed. She was starting to show symptoms of decreased urine output and irregular breathing. Instructions were given about how to position Mary and to relieve symptoms. John was tired but holding up. He slept on a cot next to Mary so he could tend to her and be with her to the end.

As death approached, both children came over and a family vigil began. On Friday night, Mary stopped eating and swallowing. Following instructions from hospice, Mary was given her morphine in concentrated form (sublingually) under her tongue. She continued to sleep most of the time. Her head up in the hospital bed, she began having periods of apnea on Sunday. At 6:00 p.m., she took her last breath with her children at the bedside. John had just left the room for a few minutes.

The hospice on-call nurse came to the house about 7:00 p.m. to help with the death. The family was sad but feeling good about having kept her at home to the end, as she had wished. John was feeling sad that he had not been with Mary at the moment she died after having cared for her so long. The nurse told him that it was very common for people to die when their spouse was not there. It was almost as if they could not leave while in the presence of the one they were most close to. This was a relief for John.

The on-call nurse arranged for the funeral home to pick up the body and helped everyone to talk about what had happened. The funeral had been planned and was arranged for the following Wednesday. The hospice chaplain had been asked to officiate. The hospice nurse and social worker came to pay respects. Mary had helped plan the event, including picking one of her favorite readings.

A few weeks passed. Family and friends began to call less often. John began to feel lonely. He did not want to burden others with the many conflicting feelings he had. About a month after Mary's death, a hospice bereavement volunteer called to introduce himself. He had a long talk with John about the events surrounding Mary's death. They agreed to get together in a few weeks. Over the next 15 months, they talked and met eight times to revisit the events surrounding Mary's life and death. John received information about grief every other month from the hospice. He came to the hospice's grief support group and met another widower about his age. They became friends and reminisced about their wives. He knew the anniversary of Mary's death would be hard. He planned a family gathering with the children and grandchildren. They all talked about Mary and how much they missed her. They had dinner and enjoyed each other's company. Mary lived on in their lives.

This chapter gave a general overview of hospice. In the next chapter, the hospice team, the foundation of hospice practice, is described in detail.

RECOMMENDED READING

Beresford, L. (1993). *The hospice handbook: A complete guide*. Boston: Little, Brown.

Byock, I. (1997). *Dying well*. New York: Putnam.

Corr, C., & Corr, D. (1983). *Hospice care: Principles and practice*. New York: Springer.

Davidson, G. (1985). *The hospice: Development and administration* (2nd ed.). Washington, DC: Hemisphere.

Jaffe, C., & Ehrlich, C. (1997). *All kinds of love: Experiencing hospice*. Amityville, NY: Baywood.

Lattanzi-Licht, M., Mahoney, J. J., & Miller, G. W. (In press, 1998). *The hospice choice: In pursuit of a peaceful death*. New York: Firestone, Simon & Schuster.

National Hospice Organization. (1993). *Standards of a hospice program of care*. Arlington, VA: NHO.

Paradis, L. F. (1985). *Hospice handbook: A guide for managers and planners*. Rockville, MD: Aspen.

Saunders, C., & Kastenbaum, R. (1997). *Hospice care on the international scene*. New York: Springer Publishing Co.

Stoddard, S. (1992). *The hospice movement: A better way of caring for the dying* (Rev. ed.). New York: Vintage Books.

Chapter Two

The Team

"If they don't have scars, they haven't worked on a team"

—Balfour Mount

THE TEAM CONCEPT

Hospice care is delivered by an interdisciplinary team. Unlike most health care settings in which there is a hierarchical structure, hospices consider all team members' input to have equal value. For a given patient and family, one team member may develop the closest relationship. It may be the home health aide, the chaplain, the physician, the social worker, the nurse, or the volunteer in whom the patient confides the most. Each patient and family served is a unique collection of life histories that combines to face death in a different way. To understand how best to treat each patient–family unit requires many different perspectives.

UNIDISCIPLINARY TO TRANSDISCIPLINARY TEAMS

To understand teams, let us explore the progression of team dynamics. First, there is the unidisciplinary team. This is a team made up of individuals who are all of the same discipline (imagine a setting where there all are social workers or engineers). In this instance, there is a collection of individuals, and everyone performs the same function. There is little team dynamic in that each is responsible for the same activity. There may be advice and consultation, but not much team interaction.

The second team concept is the multidisciplinary team. In this instance, there are people of different disciplines who work together toward a common purpose, but each has a distinct area of responsibility and works independently. Most health care settings function in this way. The interaction is usually hierarchical in that the most important discipline takes the lead. In health care, physicians take the top rung and are usually in charge and determine how care is to be delivered.

In home health care, it is the physician who orders all care and technically directs the care, even though it is usually the nurses who set everything up for the physician to approve. There is little interaction among the disciplines, and the job of each is clearly defined. Many hospices operate on a de facto multidisciplinary model.

The preferred model for hospice is the interdisciplinary model. In this approach, hierarchy is less important. There is interaction among the disciplines. Each adds to the picture of the whole patient. An interdisciplinary team values the input of all members. There are boundaries as to what each member is expected to do and focus on, but there is some blurring of boundaries. The nurse pays attention to psychosocial concerns, and the social worker attends to how symptoms may be affecting the person's ability to meet emotional needs. The home health aide may be the one the patient wants to pray with and the chaplain may hear about the family's financial concerns.

All of this is part of the flux of how families face death. Hospice may do its best work when it avoids being rigid and attends to the needs of the moment. This is not to say that it is OK to violate law or regulation or to go outside one's area of expertise. It would not work for the social worker to try to change a patient's medication dosage or for the nurse to try to do in-depth psychotherapy. Some boundaries are necessary for the safety of the patient and family.

This discussion does move toward the area of the transdisciplinary team, in which there is no hierarchical structure, and each team member acts for the patient by accessing whatever the patient and family need at the time and each member is part of a whole, be they volunteer, physician, or housekeeper.

NURSES

Nurses could be thought of as the backbone of hospice. This is meant in the true anatomical sense: They keep all parts of hospice moving. Nurses often function as case managers in hospice. In this, they are responsible for making sure all disciplines and activities are moving in the right direction. Without nurses, there would be no good symptom management, there would be no coordination of care, there would be little education and preparation for patients and families—there really would be no patient care!

Nursing is the principal means of delivering patient care in hospice. Without nurses, there would be no hospice care. So what is it that hospice nurses do? The principal activities of hospice nursing can be described as educating, treating, and managing.

The largest single activity hospice nurses perform is education. In hospice, caregivers are encouraged and empowered to do as much as possible for the patient and often more than they thought possible. Hospice nurses show families and caregivers how to provide hands-on patient care. They provide a road map for them on what to expect as the disease progresses and what to do. This removes fear and uncertainty and allows those caring to stay involved up until death. After death, those who were able to provide care have an easier time grieving. Hands-on contact with the dying person alleviates feelings of guilt and makes the experience of the patient's death more visceral and real.

Examples of educational interventions include teaching about

- administration of medications orally, rectally, or parenterally
- management of bleeding
- catheter care
- colostomy irrigation
- management of constipation
- management of dehydration
- diarrhea
- elevated temperature
- enteral feedings
- infection control
- mouth care
- pain management
- nausea
- oral and nasopharyngeal suction
- oxygen therapy and safety
- relaxation
- respiratory care
- seizure precautions
- safety
- signs and symptoms of approaching death
- skin care
- tracheostomy care

Hospice nurses treat patients. Treatments for dying patients vary widely but are generally focused on relieving distressing symptoms. All treatments are based on accurate assessment. Good hospice nurses have learned to do in-depth assessments of patients' needs. Examples of hospice nursing procedures, in addition to the above, include dressing changes, administering medication, collection of specimens, enemas, colostomy irrigation, tube insertions, impaction removal, equipment management, and postmortem care.

Hospice nurses are usually case managers. They are responsible for making sure that all disciplines are involved and meeting the patient's needs. They are responsible for developing the largest part of the care plan. They are the link to the patient's primary care physician, seeing that all orders for care are obtained. The hospice nurse works with the social worker to make sure all psychological and social concerns are addressed. She or he works with the chaplain to see that all spiritual concerns are being responded to. The nurse supervises the home health aide providing personal care and hears from the volunteer about support needs.

Hospice nurses see that the durable medical equipment the patient needs is ordered and delivered. They bring out or order all medical supplies needed, including eggcrate mattresses, adult diapers, dressings, catheters, and so forth. When medications are needed, they arrange for them to be provided. If the patient needs hospitalization for respite or symptom management, the nurses arrange for transportation and admission, prepare a transfer summary, and give a report to the facility. They visit the patient when he or she is hospitalized and continue the hospice plan of care during the inpatient stay.

Each weekday evening and all weekends and holidays, a nurse is on call to give after-hour medical advice and to make home visits as necessary. Any hospice patient and family that has a question or problem can reach a hospice nurse to discuss it 24 hours a day. Most problems can be resolved over the phone, but a substantial number require a nurse to visit. These visits can be for a leaky catheter, a patient near death or who has just died, a suddenly agitated patient, or one who is having a seizure or pain out of control. It does not matter that it may be 2:00 a.m., hospice nurses know that when the need arises, they must respond.

SOCIAL WORKERS

Facing death has a profound psychological impact on the family. The person dying gradually confronts the loss of everything. Good hospice care is distinguished by a recognition of the psychological and social needs of patients and their families. Hospices in the United States have responded to these needs mainly through provision of social work services. The hospice social worker is the primary emotional support person for the patient and family. He or she functions as both counselor and practical guide to the dying process.

On the practical side, hospice social workers help arrange for community resources that may help everyone cope better. For example, if Meals on Wheels or help from a food bank is needed, they arrange for it. If insurance coverage is confusing, they straighten it out. If the phone is disconnected, they are the patient's advocate to see it gets turned back on. If respite is needed, a volunteer or short inpatient stay is arranged. When it's time to leave the hospital, the social worker helps to do the discharge planning. Social workers help patients and families to face the difficult decisions about discontinuation of treatment and life support, funeral planning, and estate planning.

On the counseling side, the hospice social worker can go as far as the patient and family wish. Some families are severely disrupted and require in-the-home family therapy. Most everyone needs to ventilate feelings that often are unacceptable to express. The social worker is an outsider who can share the burden. A nonthreatening way for the patient to help begin to deal with his or her impending loss is to do life review. The social worker can help the patient to do an oral history of his or her life, which includes important milestones in the family, values or beliefs that ought to be passed down, instructions for survivors, and genealogical information. The process of doing this often helps the patient to gain perspective on life and to find meaning. It also helps identify any unfinished business the patient may want to attend to before death—things that need to be said to others, like "I'm sorry" or "I love you."

Providing counseling or emotional support can be done by any of the hospice disciplines, and in some programs counselors, psychologists, psychiatric nurses, or others may provide these services. The advantage of using social workers is that they can provide the needed case and resource management services along with psychological skills. In effect, one gets two services for the price of one. Social work has become a vital part of the hospice team.

PHYSICIANS

The physician member of the hospice team is most often the patient's attending physician. As a team member, he or she helps formulate and approve the patient's plan of care. The physician approves all orders and helps to achieve symptom management. Along with the hospice medical director, the physician is responsible for determining the patient's prognosis.

The relationship of the patient's physician to the hospice team varies greatly. Some physicians work in a very collaborative fashion, and others resist input and insist on controlling all aspects of care. The degree of cooperation depends on the physician's practice patterns and on his or her experience using hospice services. If the doctor adopts a unidisciplinary approach to practice, there is little room for collaboration. Most physicians being trained today have learned to appreciate the multidisciplinary approach, and some even understand interdisciplinary care.

If the physician's experience with hospice has been positive, he or she is more likely to refer and to trust hospice staff input. If hospice workers demonstrate professionalism and their recommendations result in better patient care, most physicians can be won over. Because doctors are responsible for any order they approve, they must have a high level of trust to sign off. As this trust level builds, they appreciate that hospice can shoulder much of the burdens of caring for a dying patient.

After approving a patient's entry into hospice, the attending physician may not see the patient as often. The hospice staff become the physician's eyes and ears. They report any change in condition and give periodic updates. The hospice plan of care is reviewed and approved periodically. If there is an unresolved problem or symptom, the patient is sent in for an office appointment or sometimes directly admitted to the hospital for more extensive treatment. All efforts and diagnostics are aimed at symptom relief.

The hospice medical director works in concert with the attending physician. In almost all cases, the medical director does not take over the patient's care. Exceptions to this are when the attending physician asks for hospice to provide all physician services, when there is no other physician to direct the patient's care, or when the patient requests hospice to provide attending physician services.

Hospices prefer to work with other community physicians in caring for their patients. If hospice took over the physician care, this could threaten the medical community, and there would be little opportunity for hospice to educate community physicians about palliative care.

The hospice medical director usually serves as a consultant to the medical community. If there is a problem with the way care is being managed, the medical director can intercede for the hospice staff to help correct the situation. Most attending physicians will not make home visits, and hospice patients often cannot travel comfortably. The hospice medical director can see the patient at home and give treatment recommendations to the attending physician.

The primary role of the medical director is to oversee the medical care of all hospice patients and the hospice staff's provision of clinical care. This includes providing education for hospice staff on palliative care and being a resource at all interdisciplinary team meetings. The medical director's role extends into review of all clinical policies, procedures, and protocols. There is even a role as part of the hospice's marketing efforts. Community physicians should know that the medical director is involved in the supervision of hospice staff and will ensure that the highest quality of care is being delivered. If they are respected by the local medical community, they will encourage physicians to use hospice to care for their dying patients.

HOME HEALTH AIDES

Home health aides play a critical role in hospice care. The aide is especially valued by the patient's family. Of all the disciplines in hospice, aides provide probably the most tangible assistance. It is the aide's job to provide personal care to the patient. This includes bathing, feeding, and grooming patients who are too weak or ill to care for themselves.

The family also helps with personal care, but the aide helps lift some of this burden from them. Often it is uncomfortable for grown children to provide care that is personal and intimate to a parent. Elderly spouses also are often debilitated and stressed and appreciate the aide's assistance.

In addition to personal care, the aide can assist with some nursing functions under the nurse's supervision. Aides give enemas to constipated patients, replace simple dressings, do range-of-motion exercises, assist with transferring the patient, give suppositories, give massage, provide skin care, and provide reassurance and emotional support. They report changes in condition to the nurse and reinforce education.

In hospice, the aide can also assist with some homemaker chore services. If needed, the aide can help with laundry, light housekeeping, cooking, and errands. Aides become almost a part of the family if they are able to be involved very long. For some patients, the personal and physical nature of the aide's work allows them to share some of their most intimate thoughts and feelings. The best hospice aides are those who are able to share more of themselves than their labor.

CHAPLAINS

Providing for the spiritual needs of dying patients has long been one of the facets of hospice care that has set it apart from other health care providers. Facing death inherently means facing issues of meaning and transcendence. People strive to understand what their lives have meant and what comes next after life. They agonize over past transgressions and seek forgiveness. They may seek to solidify their faith and to be more acceptable to God. They may hope to find a faith that has eluded them throughout life or to embrace a philosophical or existential position that is an expression of their being.

Whatever the struggle, hospice spiritual support staff are there to help walk with the patient or family. Hospice has always framed this as more than a question of religion. Certainly hospice is available to help with religious services. If the patient wants to pray or get in contact with a priest, minister, or rabbi for religious services, it is taken care of. What distinguishes hospice is its willingness to broaden this opportunity to include any spiritual concern. Hospice then is nondenominational in its approach to questions of meaning and the transcendent. Hospices may use a Baptist minister or a Catholic sister to respond to spiritual needs, but they all respond to the person and set aside their denominational role.

Chaplain services vary considerably among different hospices. Some programs have no one on staff but assign someone, often a social worker, to coordinate with community clergy. Others have a cadre of staff chaplains of a variety of faiths. Each hospice patient and family must have their need for spiritual support assessed by someone who is competent to evaluate. This assessment needs to address not only history of religious affiliations but the presence of common spiritual concerns such as guilt, fear of death, anger at God, estrangement, and fundamentally how they see themselves in relation to a higher power (if at all). The hospice must be capable of responding to any spiritual need identified in the assessment.

One of the difficult issues faced by hospice chaplains is providing service without being intrusive. Many times patients are unaware that they are dealing with a spiritual problem or that there is potential for spiritual growth as death nears. If the chaplain is too aggressive in presenting this to the patient, it is easy to turn the patient off. Certainly, one does not want to force any religious discussion on a patient who does not want it. The worst outcome would be if the patient were made to feel bad as a result of the intervention. Proselytizing is not condoned in hospice care. The chaplain meets the patient where he or she is and tries to offer them support and opportunities. If the patient chooses to take advantage of what the chaplain has to offer and invites the chaplain into his or her spiritual life, then the care hospice provides is richer.

Families also struggle with spiritual concerns. Many are angry at God for taking their loved one. Others are faced for the first time with their own mortality and need to sort out their spiritual beliefs. Facing death offers the patient and family an opportunity to bring their spiritual or philosophical issues into focus.

COUNSELORS

The role of counseling in hospice needs to be highlighted even though it is not the exclusive responsibility of any one discipline. In fact, all disciplines have a role in counseling the patient and family. By counseling, I mean the provision of education and emotional support. It is the giving of guidance or advice through an exchange of opinions and ideas. There are many misconceptions about terminal illness and death. Facing death is a frightening prospect for most patients and families. Usually the more information they have, the better they are able to cope. Hospice workers accept as a major charge the provision of education. Families who are prepared for the symptoms surrounding death feel more in control and confident in their caregiving.

Often, more is needed than education and support. Hospice workers may need to plan interventions that help patients and families to overcome problems or maladaptive coping. These interventions can be as simple as a relaxation exercise or as complex as having the whole team apply different strategies for each family member. Current mental health treatment offers many different tools that can help hospice workers in doing short-term counseling and intervention. For example, solutions therapy can help families focus on how they have overcome other obstacles and draw on their adaptive resources.

Various forms of family therapy are often used in hospice programs to help families cope. Hospice psychosocial assessments often include a genogram, which usually shows a three-generational description of a family including births, deaths, divorces, or other family allegiances and rivalries. How people handle death in a family is often colored by multigenerational factors. For an in-depth account of family therapy for families facing terminal illness, see *Families Facing Death* (Rosen, 1990).

Discussion of patient care, symptom management, and the dying process is likely to arouse strong feelings that also need expression. Hospice workers provide emotional support during the process of preparing the patient and family for death. They have to be sensitive to how much the family can absorb without becoming overwhelmed. The last thing anyone wants is for the patient or family to be forced to deal with painful facts they are unprepared for and then to receive no help with their emotional responses.

This is not an uncommon scenario in the health care system. What distinguishes hospice is sensitivity to these issues. Good hospice practice always involves meeting the patient and family where they are in their readiness to hear information. Hospice workers never want to beat people over the head with information. They would not want to be accused of being full of doom and gloom. Rather, hospice workers want families to eagerly anticipate their visits. Some families make it clear that they never want to discuss dying. Others are eager for any and all information about the process.

The ability to understand where the patient and family are in their desire for education and support is crucial to good hospice care. Hospice workers must be very adept at this assessment and empathetic to the emotional state of the patient and family.

The role of counseling is most often associated with the team's social worker. Social workers are responsible for assessing the family system, including levels of emotional distress and coping styles. They have much information to impart and are often the ones to address painful issues such as treatment wishes, advanced directives, and funeral planning. Nurses also play a prominent role in counseling.

It is the nurse who does the teaching of physical care and signs and symptoms of approaching death. Nurses view counseling as a major intervention, and many nursing diagnoses include correcting knowledge deficits. As an extension of the nurse, the home health aide is often called on to provide emotional support as the patient or family processes the information and emotion surrounding death.

Hospice chaplains, of course, mainly provide counseling around the spiritual aspects of facing death. Sometimes other team members are also called on to provide spiritual support. The aide or nurse may be asked to pray with the patient or the volunteer may discuss spiritual pain. Hospice provides bereavement follow-up for at least a year after the death of the patient. A bereavement counselor is available at hospice to coordinate all bereavement efforts. Some of this counseling may be provided by volunteers. The hospice staff usually does some initial bereavement visits right after the patient's death, including attendance at funerals, wakes, and so forth. This allows them to say good-bye to the family. For difficult bereavement reactions, the bereavement counselor is available, and the hospice must have access to a mental health professional who can respond to situations where pathological grief is present. Whatever the need hospice workers must be prepared to face many of life's most difficult questions.

VOLUNTEERS

In the United States, the hospice movement was founded by volunteers. All those who labored to create the first hospices did so on a volunteer basis. There were no reimbursement or funding sources. All who labored to start hospice did so because they believed that care of the dying had to be improved and that hospice was the way to do it.

Many social movements started by volunteers changed when funding became available. Services were provided by professionals, and the volunteers were brushed aside. This has happened to some degree in hospice in that volunteers have stopped functioning in most professional roles. However the role of the volunteer in U.S. hospices remains an essential one. The use of volunteers in hospice adds a major dimension to the way care is perceived by patients and families.

Paid caregivers are greatly valued, but they are in the role of employee. Volunteers are there to help because they choose to give service selflessly. Patients and families who accept the help of volunteers experience this as a higher level of human activity. Volunteers are often people who have learned from their loss experiences and choose to give back something to others. Volunteers help transform hospice into a community service rather than just a health care provider.

Volunteers are used in many roles in hospice. The primary role is in serving patients and families. Patient care volunteers usually provide support in the form of practical assistance. They help by sitting with the patient while the family goes out and being a substitute primary caregiver. They can do just about anything to help, including errands, homemaker assistance, babysitting, massage, transport, and so forth. They always are a source of emotional support to all. Some hospices use volunteers in professional roles and some are still run by volunteers.

Volunteers usually spend a block of time at least once a week at the patient's home. They can spend a great deal of time helping and often have the time to really get to know the family. Many times people will share things with their volunteer that they might not share with others because the volunteer is seen as nonthreatening.

Lay volunteers are usually taught how to handle basic patient care needs such as how to safely transfer or toilet the patient, how to give assistance when other staff are rendering care, and how to identify problems that need to be reported to the medical staff. They receive training in communication and principles of hospice and palliative care. A volunteer coordinator is usually on the staff to coordinate the efforts of volunteers. The coordinator attends team meetings, receives volunteer requests, makes assignments, supervises, and trains the volunteers.

Volunteers are used in many other ways in hospice. Ongoing bereavement support for most families can be provided by volunteers who call, visit with, and send written materials to bereaved families during the year after the death. They also help provide office assistance in hospice and help with fundraising and other community projects. Volunteers continue to be an essential part of the hospice team and are one of the components of care that distinguishes hospice care from other forms of care.

THERAPISTS

Although not part of the hospice's core team, there are a number of other disciplines that round out the group. The most prominent of the therapies are the physical, occupational, speech, respiratory, music, art (expressive), and massage therapists. The first four specialists are usually available on contract to the hospice. Because their services are usually focused on rehabilitation and hospice patients are declining, they are not used frequently.

Physical Therapist

The physical therapist is the most commonly used type of therapist. Physical therapists help patients who have difficulty ambulating or transferring. They help teach patients and families how best to move the patient and try to help maintain muscle strength through range-of-motion exercises. Patients with basic needs can be taught by the nurse. Patients with complex problems or fractures can benefit from physical therapist help in using special equipment if they are likely to live for some time.

Occupational, Speech, Respiratory, and Enterostomal Therapists

Occupational therapy can help debilitated patients continue to function longer. When used in hospice, occupational therapists teach the patient and family to use special devices so the patient can continue to eat and provide personal care longer. The speech therapist is used in hospice to assist patients who have trouble communicating. A patient who has a brain tumor or lesion who has lost speech or has other aphasic symptoms can use a speech therapist to regain some ability to communicate with family. The respiratory therapist administers breathing treatments to patients who have difficulty breathing. In addition, an enterostomal therapist can be very helpful in solving problems with stomas and are expert in skin care management.

Expressive Therapists

The art and music or expressive therapists most often work with children. They help them to express feelings that they may be unable to verbalize. This may also help create an environment for the dying person that is conducive to growth.

Massage and Pet Therapists

Massage therapy services have grown popular in many hospices. In some programs, there is a group of massage therapy volunteers who are available to work on the patient's or family members' aches and pains. They offer an adjunct that many patients enjoy and say adds to their quality of life. In some programs, there are even volunteers who use pets for therapy. Animals are brought around to visit the patients, as they can have a beneficial effect on some.

THE PATIENT AND FAMILY

The patient and family are a critical part of the hospice team. Patients can play a significant role in their own care if they are taught how at an early enough point in their illness. The patient is also the only one who can really establish the goals of care. Hospice workers can empower the patient to guide them in all they do.

In most cases, family members actually deliver most of the care given to a dying patient. They are the ones who are there with the patient day and night while hospice workers come and go. They are usually eager to learn all they can about how to deliver care. They may need care as much as or more than the patient in order to give care. They benefit in many ways by being involved in care delivery and are really the ones who deserve the credit when things go well.

One of the really unique things about hospice care is the extent to which families are allowed to be involved in the caregiving process. Nearly anything the patient needs, the family can be taught to do. With hospice, families are able to do more than they thought possible in caring for their loved one.

THE ADMINISTRATIVE TEAM

The administrative team is often overlooked as a critical part of hospice care delivery. The office staff support the clinical staff in the areas of medical records maintenance, supply ordering and stocking, billing services, accounts receivable and payable, marketing, physician relations, public relations, secretarial services, computer operations and training, and sometimes scheduling and intake.

Without the administrative team, hospice care could not be delivered. Someone has to be there to answer the phone, to page the nurse when a crisis occurs, to keep the records straight, to bill for services so everyone gets their paychecks, to prepare the paychecks, to make sure supplies are there when needed, to help order the equipment, and so on. It works best if the office staff are seen as part of the hospice team.

Some programs use the functional unit management process or self-directed work process in which operations staff are assigned to a team or service and are accountable to that group rather than to an office supervisor. However the program is organized, it is important for office staff to realize that the clinical staff are their customers and to strive to improve their services. Clinical staff who see the office support staff as part of the hospice care delivery process and value the services provided find that everything runs more smoothly.

TEAMWORK

Now that the individual disciplines in hospice have been described, it is helpful to explore how they work together to provide interdisciplinary care. After a patient has been screened for hospice eligibility, an admission–assessment visit is usually done. Some hospices have a nurse or social worker do the admission. Assessments are done after explaining all services and obtaining informed consent.

The nurse does a complete physical assessment including all systems, activities of daily living, and a thorough pain assessment. The social worker usually does the psychosocial and spiritual assessments. These assessments lead to the creation of an interdisciplinary team care plan that guides the activities of all team members.

The interdisciplinary team plan could, for example, include goals for controlling pain, educating family, meeting the patient's personal care needs, addressing family anxiety and patient depression, and helping resolve the patient's alienation from his or her church. The hospice nurse might visit daily until pain control is achieved. The nurse could assign a home health aide to bathe the patient at home three times a week and also help do the laundry.

Simultaneously, the social worker could call a family meeting to help arrange a schedule for staying with the patient. The nurse would come to the meeting to help answer questions about care and disease progression and to lessen family anxiety. The social worker would also visit privately with the patient to lean more about depressive symptoms. With the patient's permission, the hospice chaplain contacts the patient's minister to arrange home visits.

Team collaboration often occurs in office hallways or in weekly team meetings where everyone shares their perceptions of the patient. If the patient seems most concerned with getting symptoms controlled, the nurse takes the lead. If fear of dying is causing the most distress, the chaplain may take the lead. All team members focus on the areas of greatest concern.

These then are the components of the hospice caregiving team. The next chapter reviews how the hospice team successfully manages the distressing physical symptoms of terminal illness.

RECOMMENDED READING

Chang, R. Y. (1994). *Success through teamwork: A practical guide to international team dynamics*. Irvine, CA: Chang Associates.

Katzenbaum, J. R., & Smith, D. K. (1993). *The wisdom of teams: Creating the high performance organization*. Boston, MA: Harvard Business School Press.

Larson, D. (1993). *The helper's journey: Working with people facing grief, loss, and life threatening illness*. Illinois: Research Press.

Parker, G. M. (1996). *Team players and teamwork: The new competitive business strategy*. New Jersey: Jossey-Bass.

Robbins, H., & Finley, M. (1995). *Why teams don't work: What went wrong and how to make it right*. New Jersey: Peterson's Guides.

Sanborn, M. (1995). *Teambuilt: Making team work work*. New York: Mastermedia.

Towery, T. L. (1995). *The wisdom of wolves: Nature's way to organizational success*. Indiana: Wessex House Publications.

Wellins, R. S., Byham, W. C., & Wilson, J. M. (1991). *Empowered teams: Creating self directed work groups that improve quality, productivity and participation*. New Jersey: Jossey-Bass.

Whyte, D. (1996). *The heart aroused: Poetry and Preservation of the Soul*. New York: Bantam Doubleday Dell.

Chapter Three

Symptom Management and Physical Care

If you ask people who are terminally ill what they fear most, it usually is dying, not death itself. In our culture, terminal illness is equated with suffering. To face death is to confront the knowledge that one may have to endure unimaginable distress. Perhaps this is why in some Asian cultures, it is thought preferable to withhold the truth from those found to be incurably ill.

Unfortunately, in the United States and most of the rest of the world, dying can still be an agonizing process. Either there is no knowledge of palliative medicine or there are too few resources to provide adequate care, or both. Ours is a world where to face death usually means to experience unrelieved symptoms, indignity, and the loss of all that is meaningful. It is not so surprising that people seek out a physician to provide euthanasia.

A recent report (SUPPORT Investigators, 1995) on efforts to improve care for seriously ill hospitalized patients had some troubling findings. One half of the patients who died had moderate or severe pain during their final 3 days of life. Only 41% of patients reported talking to their physicians about prognosis or cardiopulmonary resuscitation (CPR). Physicians misunderstood patient preferences regarding CPR in 80% of cases. When patients wanted CPR withheld, a do-not-resuscitate order was never written in 50% of cases.

If the hospice movement has taught us anything, it is that dying does not have to be this way. Nearly all hospice patients are free of physical pain in the time leading up to their deaths. A recent study by the NHO looked at how well pain was controlled in the last 30 days of life for hospice patients. Readings were taken from patients' reports at each nursing visit by means of a scale ranging from 0 to 10, with 0 equaling *no pain* and 10 equaling *the worst imaginable pain*. Mean scores were summed for each patient, and those means were then averaged to derive a global mean pain level for each hospice. The overall mean for the 11 hospices participating was 1.67. This meant that overall these hospices kept their patients' pain well controlled up to the time of death (NHO, 1995b).

Hospices also understand that suffering encompasses a broader sphere than pain alone. Eric Cassell (1982), in his classic article "The Nature of Suffering and the Goals of Medicine," showed that suffering can occur in different dimensions of the person. Physical distress may cause suffering or may be viewed as redemptive or as leading to a goal, as in childbirth. Cassell argued that "suffering occurs when an impending destruction of the person is perceived; it continues until the threat of disintegration has passed or until the integrity of the person can be restored in some other manner."

Hospices attempt to help patients deal with as many of the different dimensions of suffering as possible. If the patient is experiencing spiritual pain, increasing the morphine dose will not solve the problem; intervention by the chaplain may be necessary. If the patient develops neuropathic pain, supportive counseling will be less effective than adding a coanalgesic. Care of dying patients requires very careful assessment.

TRAJECTORIES OF DYING

Most cancer patients follow a fairly predictable downhill course as the disease progresses. There are increasing symptoms, and functional ability decreases. Expanding hospice care to people with different disease categories has taught hospice workers that there are differences in this expected course of events.

People in the advanced stages of AIDS follow a roller-coaster course, often with many close encounters with death. The course of AIDS continues to change as the disease manifests itself in different conditions. Whereas it was common for many people with AIDS to die after a single episode of *Pneumocystis carinii* pneumonia, there are now many who have survived numerous episodes of it. Kaposi's sarcoma used to be a much more common syndrome than it is today, and it would usually result in a fairly fast downhill demise.

New treatments for AIDS, especially the protease inhibitors, now hold promise as prolonged therapy becomes more effective. In the "Medical Guidelines for Determining Prognosis in Selected Non-Cancer Terminal Illnesses" (NHO, 1996b), it is expected that the guidelines for AIDS will have to be reexamined about every 6 months, in light of the rapidly changing treatment environment.

Even medical oncology is undergoing significant changes. Although the overall cancer death rate has not declined in recent decades, there are now many new treatments available. There have been significant improvements in the prognoses for people with Hodgkin's disease, testicular cancer, and some leukemias. Some patients with prostate cancer can look forward to such slow disease progression that they will likely die of conditions other than their cancer.

With many of the other chronic, life-threatening illnesses such as chronic obstructive pulmonary disease, congestive heart failure, and Alzheimer's disease, there are often periods of exacerbation followed by periods of stability. A patient with congestive heart failure may have many life-threatening episodes requiring hospitalization. While the person is an inpatient, medical intervention can stabilize symptoms to where the patient returns home. This cycle can repeat for years until the patient's body simply gives out or until the patient decides to let the disease run its natural course without aggressive intervention.

It is often the decision about how to treat the patient that determines if the patient is at a "terminal" stage. For many people with these chronic conditions, how exacerbations are treated determines when they are terminal. For the patient with chronic obstructive pulmonary disease, it may be the decision to forgo ventilator treatment; for the Alzheimer's patient, it may be the point when a decision is reached to not treat generalized infection. For the cancer patient, it may be when the burden of experiencing aggressive chemotherapeutic side effects outweighs the possible benefit of prolonging life.

Once this turning point is reached, the focus of care can shift to the goal of comfort. The aim is not to fight for cure of the disease but to simply live as fully as possible for as long as possible. To reach this goal, the patient must be relieved of distress. In the Maslovian (1967) view, the patient must first be free from physical pain and other symptoms such as nausea, constipation, confusion, shortness of breath, and so forth. This has to be accomplished before any psychological, emotional, social, or transcendent issues can be attended to and resolved. In this hierarchy, pain is usually attended to first.

PAIN MANAGEMENT

It is not within the scope of this work to undertake a thorough explanation of pain management. There are several excellent references for the reader who wishes to delve more deeply into the subject (see the list of recommended readings at the end of the chapter). Some of the key distinguishing factors that make the hospice approach more effective are reviewed here. Treatment of pain requires a well-developed knowledge of assessment.

The International Association for the Study of Pain defined pain as "an unpleasant sensory and emotional experience associated with actual or potential tissue damage" (Foley, 1985). Pain is always subjective; there is no way to distinguish pain occurring in the absence of tissue damage from pain resulting from tissue damage. Pain is what the patient says is pain. Caregivers must always be alert to the reality that pain is multidimensional. In addition to physical pain, there is the potential for enormous psychological, social, and spiritual pain.

The first distinction in assessment of physical pain is between chronic and acute pain. Acute pain is associated with a well-defined onset due to an external insult or internal event and results in hyperactivity of the autonomic nervous system. Chronic pain has a less well-defined temporal onset and persists for longer than 6 months. The autonomic nervous system adapts, and there are fewer objective signs. Rather, there are significant changes in personality, functional ability, and life-style that require treating not only the pain but its complications.

Hospice patients are generally faced with chronic pain from their illnesses. There are periods when hospice patients are faced with acute pain episodes related to their primary diagnosis or its treatment, but the vast majority of pain problems are chronic in nature. Although patients with noncancer terminal illnesses do experience pain, it is malignant disease that is most often associated with pain syndromes. Pain associated with cancer is primarily one of three types: somatic, visceral, or deafferentation.

Somatic, or nociceptive, pain is the most common type of cancer pain and occurs as a result of activation of nociceptors in cutaneous and deep tissues. This pain is usually well localized and constant and is often described as aching or gnawing. Painful bone metastasis is an example of somatic pain.

Visceral pain results from stretching or distending the viscera, usually as a result of metastatic tumor. This is also a common cancer pain, is not well localized, and is often described as squeezing or pressure pain. Metastatic infiltration of the liver is an example of visceral pain.

The third major type of cancer pain is deafferentation pain, which is the result of injury to the peripheral or central nervous systems, or both. This is due to tumor compression or infiltration of the nerves. It can also occur as a result of surgery, chemotherapy, or radiation (Foley, 1985). Deafferentation pain can be quite severe and is often described as a constant dull ache punctuated with episodes of burning or electrical-shock–like sensations. Examples of deafferentation pain include metastatic or treatment-induced lumbosacral or brachial plexopathies.

Proper control of pain requires an accurate assessment of the type of pain the patient experiences. Most somatic and visceral pain responds to narcotic and nonnarcotic agents. Deafferentation pain is often poorly tolerated and difficult to control. Many patients have more than one type of pain. It is critical for staff to assess each pain source carefully. Hospices use a variety of pharmacologic and psychological approaches to the management of pain.

There are several important palliative care principles that hospices apply in the treatment of chronic pain. First, for constant pain, medication must be given around the clock. If the drug is immediate-release morphine, it must be given about every 4 hours. It is more common today to use long-acting narcotics whose duration of action is 8–24 hours. This allows for less frequent dosing and avoidance of sleep interruption. Regular around-the-clock dosing is critical to controlling pain. Many cancer patients are put on an as-needed or PRN dosing of medication. This creates a vicious cycle of yo-yoing back and forth between pain relief and the return of pain. Regular use of pain medication stops this cycle and eliminates the patient's memory and fear of pain.

A second principle is to give or titrate the proper amount of medication. Some clinicians fear giving large doses of narcotics. They are usually afraid of overdosing the patient. Hospices have yet to find a ceiling to how much medication can be safely given. The art is to give enough to control the pain without causing sedation or unwanted side effects. When starting out, it is best to give enough to make sure the pain is controlled. Good pain control is not achieved by sneaking up on the pain. It is often necessary to give a significant dose increase to get on top of the pain. Once this is accomplished, the dose can be adjusted on the basis of feedback from the patient.

Another cardinal rule in controlling pain is that pain is what the patient says is pain. The only one who can accurately measure pain and pain relief is the patient. Studies of surrogate measurement of pain find that medical staff or family do not give accurate ratings of pain when compared with the patient's own ratings (Grossman, Scheidler, Swedeen, Mucenski, Piantadosi, 1991; Teske, Dant, & Cleeland, 1983). Continuous titration of the patient's medication dosage is critical to the control of pain. Hospice nurses often use a pain measurement scale, such as a simple 0–10 scale, with 0 being *pain free* and 10 being *the worst imaginable pain*. Most patients want to be pain free, but some are quite content with keeping the pain at 3 or below on this scale.

When titrating pain medication, the focus is usually on breakthrough pain. This is the pain experienced before the next dose of medication is due. When using a long-acting narcotic, there is usually a short-acting narcotic available as a supplement. When the use of the short-acting narcotic reaches a large enough dose, the dose of the long-acting narcotic is increased.

Pharmacologic treatment is often divided, using the World Health Organization (1990) analgesic ladder, into mild, moderate, and severe pain. Mild pain is treated with nonopiods with or without an adjuvant. Moderate pain is treated with an opiod for mild to moderate pain and a nonopiod analgesic, with or without an adjuvant. Severe pain is treated with an opiod for moderate to severe pain, with or without nonopiod and adjuvant treatment.

OTHER SYMPTOMS

Other symptoms that can often accompany terminal illness include nausea and vomiting, dyspnea, diarrhea and constipation, anorexia, weakness, and confusion. (For a more thorough discussion of symptom management in terminally ill persons, refer to the list of recommended readings at the end of the chapter).

Nausea and Vomiting

Nausea and vomiting occur in 60% of terminal cancer patients at some stage but tend to be intermittent (Kaye, 1993). Nausea can have numerous causes, and careful assessment is imperative. According to Kaye, the most common causes are

- drug side effects
- oral thrush
- brain metastases
- anxiety
- gastric irritation
- intestinal obstruction
- constipation
- small stomach syndrome
- hypercalcemia
- uremia
- low-grade urinary tract or pulmonary infection

Nausea usually has more than one cause and can become a conditioned response. Many different drugs can cause nausea, and it is a good idea to avoid polypharmacy. Using the right antiemetic by the appropriate route is critical. The oral route is best for prophylaxis, whereas suppositories or injections are usually needed during the first 24 hours. A continuous subcutaneous infusion may be useful for severe nausea and vomiting.

Other recommendations include use of more than one antiemetic, use of steroids or H_2 receptor antagonist, change of opioid drug, behavioral treatment, and in rare instances a celiac plexus block. Vomiting with little or no nausea can occur with high intestinal obstruction, regurgitation, or with raised intracranial pressure. Some patients can tolerate occasional vomiting if nausea is controlled.

Dyspnea

A recent review article (Pang, 1994) found the incidence of dyspnea in advanced malignancies varied from 48–78.6% of patients. Breathlessness is a frequent part of the dying process and can usually be managed with palliative measures. Shortness of breath during the course of illness can be due to multiple causes, including

- anemia
- ascites
- bronchospasm
- cardiac failure
- lung collapse
- lung infection
- pericardial effusion
- pleural effusion
- pneumothorax

- pulmonary emboli
- superior vena cava obstruction

Treatment varies, depending on the etiology of the dyspnea and condition of the patient. If the patient is far from endstage, it may make sense to treat anemia with transfusion or a lung infection with an antibiotic, whereas at endstage or in chronic breathlessness, the more conservative palliative measures would include use of morphine and ativan with relaxation therapy, reassurance, and oxygen or possibly an electric fan.

There has been some disagreement over the effectiveness of oxygen in terminal dyspnea. A recent double-blind study (Bruera, de Stoutz, Velasco-Leiva, Schoeiler, Hanson, 1993) found that oxygen was beneficial to patients with hypoxia and dyspnea when at rest.

Diarrhea and Constipation

Although these are thought of as opposites, they are often connected and are part of a continuum of gastrointestinal disturbances. Constipation is a very frequent complaint of terminally ill persons, often as a side effect of narcotic use. Kaye (1993) reported that in a study of 200 hospice patients, 75% needed rectal measures (enema or bowel protocol) within a week of admission. Other frequent causes of constipation are

- low-fiber diet
- failure to heed the urge or reduced defecation
- dehydration
- depression
- hypercalcemia

In addition to opioids, diuretics and anticholinergics can cause constipation.

The most frequent cause of constipation in terminal patients is the regular use of opioids without the concurrent use of adequate doses of laxatives. Even patients with little intake should not go more than 3 days without a bowel movement. Laxative treatment should include both a fecal softener and a stimulant laxative. Bulk-forming laxatives can be contraindicated as they may lead to impaction. Patients with impaction will need enema or manual disempaction.

Diarrhea is found in patients with impaction as small amounts of liquid feces leak past the fecal mass. Other causes of diarrhea include

- steatorrhea (due to malabsorption of fat)
- malignant intestinal obstruction
- laxative imbalance
- rectal tumor
- fecal incontinence due to loss of sphincter control or recto-vaginal fistula
- carcinoid tumor

Anorexia

Loss of appetite occurs in the majority of hospice patients as illness progresses. It is a normal consequence of disease progression and not due to poor eating habits on the patient's part, as many families seem to think. Factors contributing to anorexia include

- oral thrush
- constipation
- nausea
- hypercalcemia
- chemotherapy
- depression

Treatment of anorexia includes administration of steroids to increase appetite, attention to attractive meal preparation, and patient–family education. Generally, patients are more likely to eat if they are presented with small, more frequent meals or snacks. Attention to presentation can include use of garnish, care to avoid strong odors, concentration on bland foods, and a bit of detective work in an effort to serve meals that the patient prefers.

Education of the family is very important. They can feel rejection as the patient refuses to eat. They need to understand that taste abnormalities are common in seriously ill people, that the body need less intake when inactive, and that they can continue to give the patient whatever he or she wants, especially fluids, up until the end.

Confusion

Various changes in mental status are common in terminally ill persons. Confusion is found in about 30% of cancer patients at some point in their illness. The causes of confusion include

- drugs
- full bladder
- pain
- impaction
- brain metastases
- infection
- metabolic imbalance
- anxiety
- withdrawal from alcohol or benzodiazepines
- delirium

Most psychoactive medication can cause confusion, usually because of deterioration in liver or kidney functioning. Many other medications can cause confusion, including diuretics, beta blockers, anti-Parkinsonian drugs, and sulfonamides. As death approaches, it is not uncommon for patients to experience delirium as part of the endstage process.

One of the most difficult symptoms to manage is severe agitated confusion. In this state, the patient may become aggressive, paranoid, terrified, or greatly distressed. Immediate sedation may be needed. Families have a very hard time managing patients who are up all night trying to get out of bed without pharmaceutical intervention.

Symptom management is important to the patient's quality of life. Without good symptom management, it is difficult to have quality of life. However, having good symptom management does not ensure quality of life.

MANAGEMENT OF IMPENDING DEATH

Effective management of the symptoms found at the endstage of the illness is critical to achieving a good death. For cancer and most other chronic diseases, there is a symptom complex as death nears that has a number of distinguishing characteristics.

This cluster of symptoms usually includes lowered body temperature, increased somnolence, confusion, incontinence, congestion in the lungs or throat, restlessness, withdrawal or detachment from others, visionlike experiences, decreased intake of fluid and foods, decreased urine output, and changes in breathing.

Common interventions that help manage the symptoms of impending death are shown in the box below.

EDUCATION AND CAREGIVING

Good physical care for a dying patient is very important to comfort. Having the right medication and psychosocial support is not enough if one is lying all day in wet sheets because there is no one there to change the bed. Hospices do not usually provide around-the-clock caregivers. Either family, friends, or paid caregivers must be identified to deliver this basic care to the patient under hospice's supervision.

Some hospices offer private-duty caregivers that the patient must pay for to provide care around the clock. Under the Hospice Medicare Benefit there is also provision for continuous care during periods of crisis where hospice can send in nurses for 8–24 hours in a day. Still, the bulk of care must be provided by nonhospice caregivers.

The primary caregiver is often a spouse or other family member. This person usually has little experience caring for a seriously ill person. Hospices have developed training materials to familiarize people with how to provide basic safe

Symptom	Intervention
Coolness	Warm the patient, but not with an electric blanket.
Somnolence	A normal reaction. Sit with the patient.
Confusion	Speak softly, clearly, and truthfully.
Incontinence	Catheter, chucks, or adult diapers
Congestion in lungs or throat	Position head to the side; clear mouth or airway. Medication or suction may be used if necessary.
Restlessness	Light massage, quiet voice, soothing music
Withdrawal or detachment from others	Give space; encourage interpersonal communication to extent comfortable to person; assess for depression.
Visionlike experiences	Do not discount; ask for details. Try to understand symbolic meanings. Offer reassurance if troubled.
Decreased intake of fluid and foods	Give supplements as tolerated. Pay attention to presentation of food and fluids. Maintain good mouth care.
Decreased urine output	Monitor intake and output. Consider a foley catheter. Usually a sign that death is nearing.
Changes in breathing	Irregular breathing, periods of apnea, Cheyne-Stokes and wet respirations. Elevate the head, turn patient on side. Hold hand. Speak gently.

care. The hospice nurse or aide always demonstrates how to perform a procedure and usually gives written instruction for reference.

The kinds of procedures typically taught to hospice families include the following:

- medication administration
- catheter care
- how to handle bleeding
- dressing changes
- colostomy care
- constipation
- signs and symptoms of approaching death
- dehydration
- diarrhea

- elevated temperature
- infection control
- durable medical equipment operation
- hospital bed change
- body mechanics to avoid injury
- IV therapy
- mouth care
- nausea
- oral and nasopharyngeal suction
- oxygen safety
- relaxation
- seizure precautions
- skin care
- pericare
- tracheostomy care
- pain control

The type of teaching needed will depend on the needs of the patient. Caregivers are able to cope better the more they know about the needs of the patient. Hospice staff have to be able to assess how much a caregiver can be expected to do. Some are able to learn right away, others are too emotionally upset to learn. Sometimes the relationship precludes doing care. Many children have a difficult time with the thought of doing personal care for a parent.

Empowering caregivers to do more than they thought they could in caring for the patient is healthy. Spousal involvement in caregiving may powerfully mediate the somatic effects of grief (Connor, 1996a). There is much anecdotal experience in hospice that suggests that patients live longer if they receive competent and consistent care from a primary caregiver.

CASE ILLUSTRATION

John

John was a 56-year-old non–small cell lung cancer patient with metastatic disease to the bone who was admitted to hospice while in the hospital. He had been treated unsuccessfully with chemotherapy and wanted to return home. On admission, he was still nauseated from chemotherapy and was too weak to get out of bed without assistance. He had residual movement pain from bone metastases.

He had difficulty breathing and was on oxygen in the hospital. At hospice admission, his medications included percocet 10 mg as needed, tigan 250 mg three times a day, and IV fluids. He had not had a bowel movement in 3 days, and he rated his pain as 5 on the 0–10 scale.

He lived with his wife and two teenage sons; an older daughter lived nearby. His wife worked as a sales clerk, and up until his diagnosis 5 months earlier he had worked as a car mechanic. He was generally angry and impatient with the indignities of being in the health care system.

He was transferred to the hospice unit to prepare for discharge home. On transfer, his medications were changed to ms-contin 30 mg twice daily, naprosyn 500 mg twice daily, compazine 5 mg three times daily, and senekot-s. He was given an enema and disempacted. Hospice nurses began teaching him and his family about care in the home and what to expect.

After 24 hours, he reported that his pain was at 1 on the 0–10 scale and that his nausea was controlled. He was able to get up out of bed and had less shortness of breath. He had resisted getting up due to movement pain, and he now reported only very mild pain when ambulating. His IV was removed, and he was able to eat a diet as tolerated.

Plans for his discharge were made and he went home with his family. Before discharge, a hospital bed and an oxygen tank were delivered. He no longer needed continuous oxygen as the morphine relieved his respiratory distress; the tank was there for reassurance and for occasional use should he become short of breath. He was sent home with a supply of medication, and once there was visited by his hospice home care nurse. She assessed the home and made sure he and his family felt prepared to handle his care.

A home health aide was assigned to come the next day to help John with his personal care. The social worker and chaplain had visits scheduled during the week. On Thursday night, John's wife called the hospice on-call service because John was having an episode of anxiety. He was short of breath and could not get comfortable. The nurse on call got an order from the patient's physician for ativan 2 mg to be given twice daily. The order was called into the pharmacy and was picked up by the nurse on her way to visit the home. Within an hour of giving the ativan, John felt more comfortable. The nurse also instructed the patient in the use of a relaxation exercise to control anxiety.

John's care went smoothly for another 3 weeks until he began to develop more pain. He was started on oral morphine solution 5 mg per cc for breakthrough pain. His oral morphine solution dose gradually increased until his ms contin dose is moved to 60 mg twice daily. At first, he needed no oral morphine solution, but gradually he began to have breakthrough pain. As his pain increased, the long-acting and immediate-release doses of morphine were adjusted to stay on top of his pain.

John gradually got weaker and was confined to bed. As death approached, he began to have trouble swallowing. His ms-contin dose was put into small gelatin capsules, and his family was taught how to give them rectally. He was able to take liquids and ice chips. He died peacefully at home with his wife and three children at his side. The hospice nurse came to the house and called the funeral home. She complimented the family on the care they were able to give John and they talked about how life would be without him. She reminded them of the bereavement support services available for the next year, and the funeral home arrived to take John's body.

Once the physical symptoms of terminal illness are under control, it is possible to begin to deal with psychological and spiritual concerns. In the next chapter, some of the more common psychosocial and spiritual concerns of the dying are addressed.

RECOMMENDED READING

Amenta, M. O., & Bohnet, N. (1986). *Nursing care of the terminally ill*. Boston: Little, Brown.

Billings, J. A. (1985). *Outpatient management of advanced cancer: Symptom control, support and hospice in-the-home*. Philadelphia: Lippincott.

Blues, A., & Zerwekh, J. (1984). *Hospice and palliative nursing care*. New York: Grune & Stratton.

Doyle, D., Hanks, G., & McDonald, N. (Eds.). (1993). *Oxford textbook of palliative medicine*. New York: Oxford University Press.

Kaye, P. (1993). *Notes on symptom control in hospice and palliative care*. Essex, CT: Hospice Education Institute.

McCaffery, M. (1979). *Nursing management of the patient with pain*. Philadelphia: Lippincott.

Petrosino, B. (1986). *Nursing in hospice and terminal care: Research and practice*. New York: Hayworth Press.

Woodruff, R. (1996). *Palliative medicine: Symptomatic and supportive care for patients with advanced cancer and AIDS*. Melbourne, Victoria, Australia: Asperula.

Chapter Four

Psychosocial and Spiritual Care

"The more complete one's life is, the more . . . one's creative capacities are fulfilled, the less one fears death . . . People are not afraid of death per se, but of the incompleteness of their lives."

—Lisl Marburg Goodman

The knowledge of impending death has profound psychological and social impact on human beings. Humans are the only animals who know their own mortality. In an attempt to understand how humans cope with this knowledge, some have attempted to develop theories that give a road map for how to prepare for death.

The psychological and spiritual aspects of coping with impending death are intertwined. It is an arena where psychology and religion overlap. How people cope emotionally is affected by their spiritual belief system, and their capacity for spiritual growth is influenced by psychological health.

REACTIONS TO THE KNOWLEDGE OF IMMINENT DEATH

Death defines life. It gives people's lives meaning and context, yet nothing is as feared or as assiduously avoided. There are probably as many reactions to dying as there are people who die. It is intriguing how individuals faced with comparable tragedies can respond so differently. One person may be incapacitated with anxiety and dread; another reacts with stoic resignation. Recently, a patient said he felt that "death was a big present with a bow on it." He couldn't wait to find out what was inside.

Weisman (1972) originated the concept of "appropriate death." He described this as a purposeful death. Appropriate death should be pain free with emotional and social impoverishments kept to a minimum. The person should be able to function as effectively as possible as long as possible before dying. Conflicts should be recognized and resolved, and remaining wishes should be satisfied. Control should be yielded to others in whom the dying person has confidence. However, what might be an appropriate death for one person might be unsuitable for another.

A considerable body of research has pointed to the view that in adults, age is negatively correlated with fear of death. Bengston, Ceullar, and Ragan (1977) studied three age groups: 45–55, 55–64, and 65–74 years. The youngest cohort expressed the most fear of death, whereas the oldest expressed the least. Similar results were found by Kalish and Reynolds (1977), Wass (1977), Devins (1979), Cappon (1978), and Kastenbaum and Aisenberg (1972).

A number of factors account for this tendency. Elderly people are more often confronted with death among their peers. Death is viewed culturally as the natural conclusion to the life cycle. Older persons are more likely to believe in an afterlife (Kalish & Reynolds, 1977). They may be less concerned about survivors and less concerned about having additional life experiences.

Is it true that people die as they lived? In the sense that people cope with death the way they have coped with other problems in life, perhaps yes. Yet there are times when the dying process inflicts indignities that seem so inappropriate to a loving, caring person or when death seems so easy for the hard hearted.

People's responses to the knowledge of impending death are not linear. They are characterized by vacillations in emotional and cognitive responses. Most often the human reaction is that of ambivalence—the coexistence of fearful avoidance and the desire for release.

Rather than being contradictory, ambivalence seems a natural part of the dying process. Death as the ultimate unknown is usually feared. Underneath people's managed exterior is a raw terror of annihilation. In life, people attempt to control events; at the moment of death, control is gone. In juxtaposition to fear, many grow weary of the struggle to stay alive. They may also be curious as to what lies ahead. At times, death may also be seen as a solution to life's unanswered questions.

STAGE THEORY

People have a great need for landmarks and labels when dealing with the mysteries of the dying process. They feel more comfortable and less helpless if there is a predictable road map to follow. This may explain why Elisabeth Kübler-Ross's (1969) five stages of dying (denial, anger, depression, bargaining, and acceptance) became so universally accepted as *the* explanation of the dying process.

As a metaphor for dealing with all losses, Kübler-Ross's (1969) theory seems to fit with human experience. She provided a new language that can be useful if not used too concretely. Kastenbaum (1974) stated that the problems with stage theories of dying are that they reckon little with the symptoms and trajectories of a particular disease state, with the person's personality, or with the person's environment. He also criticized the lack of any scientific evidence for the five stages (Kastenbaum & Kastenbaum, 1989).

Garfield (1978) challenged the notion that all people—regardless of belief system, age, race, culture, and historical period—die in a uniform sequence. Kalish (1978) questioned whether all patients go through stages and highlighted the influence of the medical care system on the patient's reactions to illness. The goals of cure and rehabilitation can encourage reactions such as denial and anger.

Dying persons show a variety of emotions that ebb and flow throughout their lives. These emotional reactions or stages can vary from minute to minute. A wide variety of emotions are seen in dying people, some displaying a few, some a great many. Instead of defining a universal, sequential order of stages of dying, it may be more helpful to describe phases of dying and courses of illness that demand different coping strategies at different times.

Holland (1989) described several possible courses for the patient following a cancer diagnosis:

- treatment leading to long survival and cure
- treatment leading to survival with no evidence of disease, followed by recurrence
- treatment with poor response and no disease-free interval, followed by palliative treatment and death
- no primary treatment possible, followed by palliative treatment and death

For the patient who experiences many remissions, there may be considerable uncertainty, ambiguity, and several episodes of heightened anxiety and preparation for death. There is also uncertainty as to length of remission (or "cure") and when recurrence will occur.

Another view of the phases involved in dying of a terminal illness was offered by Weisman (Pattison, 1978). These include

- the acute crisis-of-knowledge phase
- the chronic, living–dying interval (middle knowledge)
- the terminal phase

Weisman added that, given the same disease, people do not follow the same sequence and do not die at the same rate, of the same causes, or in the same circumstances. There is no well-recognized succession of emotional responses that are typical of people facing death. Pattison (1978) believed that the concept of stages of dying is not only inaccurate but misleading to both the dying person and his or her helpers. There are no typical deaths. Dying may be stageless.

PSYCHOSOCIAL CARE OF DYING PERSONS AND THEIR FAMILIES

The International Work Group (IWG) on Death, Dying, and Bereavement is a voluntary nonprofit organization composed of recognized leaders in the field. The group was formed in 1974 to help promote and advance the understanding of the needs of dying persons and their families. The group meets at approximately 18-month intervals to advance knowledge in the field and to develop consensus documents on important areas of concern in the care of dying patients and their families. These IWG documents are usually statements of assumptions and principles.

IWG documents have been produced on terminal care, ethics, bereavement, care of the dying and bereaved in developing countries, spiritual care, education, HIV, palliative care for children, death and the arts, research and practice, and violence.

A "Statement of Assumptions and Principles Concerning Psychosocial Care of Dying Persons and Their Families" was developed in a work group I chaired (International Work Group on Death, Dying, and Bereavement, 1993). These assumptions and principles address the important psychosocial issues facing the dying, their families, and caregivers and offer advice about handling them. They are reprinted here for the reader's reference:[1]

Introduction

The dying and their families face numerous psychosocial issues as death approaches. In writing the following assumptions and principles concerning these issues we hope to counteract the tendency to focus too much on physical and technical care, to stimulate readers to test the following assumptions against their own experience, and to incorporate them into their work.

By psychosocial we mean the emotional, intellectual, spiritual, interpersonal, social, cultural, and economic dimensions of the human experience. Assumptions and principles for spiritual care have been developed by other work groups of the IWG.

[1]Developed by the Psychosocial Work Group of the IWG: Dr. Thelma Bates (United Kingdom), Rev. David Head (United Kingdom), Ms. Constance Connor (United States), Ms. Shirley Henen (South Africa), Dr. Stephen Connor (United States), Dr. Isa Jaramillo (Colombia), Ms. Donna Corr (United States), Dr. Scott Long (United States), Ms. Esther Gjertsen (Norway), and Dr. Colin M. Parkes (United Kingdom).

By family we mean those individuals who are part of the dying person's most immediate attachment network, regardless of blood or matrimonial ties. The family, which includes the dying person, is the unit of care. By caregivers we mean those professionals and volunteers who provide care to dying persons and their families. We have separated the dying person, the family, and caregivers for the purpose of discussion only. Many of these assumptions and principles apply equally to dying persons and their families. They may not apply to all cultures and belief systems.

Issues for Dying Persons

ASSUMPTIONS	PRINCIPLES
1. Dying persons may choose to acknowledge or not acknowledge their impending death.	1. Caregivers must recognize and respect the person's right to deny or not communicate about his or her impending death. Caregivers may be helpful to family members and others in understanding or accepting the dying person's position, which may change with time.
2. Dying persons can communicate about their impending death in different cultural ways, encompassing verbal, nonverbal, or symbolic ways of communicating.	2. Caregivers must seek understanding and knowledge of the dying person's cultural and life-style experiences. Caregivers need to be astutely sensitive to nonverbal and symbolic ways of communicating and recognize that these modalities may be more significant to the dying person than verbal expression.
3. Dying persons have the right to information on their changing physical status, and the right to choose whether or not to be told they are dying.	3. Caregivers need to be sensitive and perceptive to the different ways the person may be requesting information about his or her condition.
4. Dying persons may be preoccupied with dying, death itself, or with what happens after death.	4. The caregiving team needs to be aware of the dying person's concerns and fears in order to provide care that is responsive and supportive.

5. Dying persons can have a deep-seated fear of abandonment. They may therefore continue treatment for the sake of the family or physician rather than in the belief that it will be of personal benefit.

5. Caregivers can be helpful to the dying person in identifying feelings that may affect treatment decisions.

Caregivers may also be helpful in opening communication between the dying patient and family or physician that may clearly reflect the patient's goal for treatment.

6. Many dying persons experience multiple physical and psychological losses before their death.

6. Caregivers may be helpful in facilitating the expression of grief related to the multiple losses of terminal illness. Caregivers may also be helpful in supporting the dying person's need for continued autonomy, satisfying roles and activities, and meaning despite these losses.

7. Dying persons exhibit a variety of coping strategies in facing death.

7. Caregivers need to be able to recognize the utility of adaptive coping mechanisms and be tolerant of the patient's or families' need to use or abandon such mechanisms. Caregivers can help to foster an environment that encourages the use of effective ways of coping by accurately addressing the dying persons' concern.

8. Dying persons generally need to express feelings.

8. Dying persons should not be isolated but given the opportunity to communicate.

9. Dying persons communicate when they feel safe and secure.

9. Caregivers should strive to create an environment in which communication can be facilitated, paying special attention to physical comfort, symptom management, physical surroundings, privacy, confidentiality, adequate time, acceptance of feelings, and shared expectations.

10. Dying persons may find it helpful to communicate with others who are terminally ill.

10. Opportunities should be encouraged for patient interaction such as peer or professionally facilitated support groups, social functions, or designated areas within treatment settings where patients may informally gather.

11. A dying person's communication of concern about death may be inhibited by a number of psychosocial and culturally determined expectations.

11. Caregivers can be helpful in breaking through the barriers that inhibit the dying person's true expression of feelings.

12. Dying persons have a right to be acknowledged as living human beings until their death.

12. Even when they seem severely impaired, dying persons are still able to sense their own surroundings. Caregivers need to facilitate this awareness. Caregivers should encourage behavior, touch, and communication, which continue to demonstrate respect for the dying person.

13. Dying persons' psychological suffering may be greater than their physical pain or discomfort.

13. Caregivers should recognize, and attend to, the psychological component of suffering.

14. Dying persons may have difficulty in dealing with the different or conflicting needs of family members.

14. Caregivers need to be aware of the dynamics within each family and recognize the importance of dealing with individual members as well as the family unit. Caregivers should be sensitive to the presence of conflicts between family members, and may need to maintain a position of neutrality in order to be effective.

Issues for Families

ASSUMPTIONS	PRINCIPLES
1. Families have fundamental needs to care and be cared for.	1. Families should be encouraged to provide whatever care they can. Caregivers should not supplant the family in the caregiver role except where the family lacks physical or emotional resources, knowledge, or desire to provide care. By providing care to family members, caregivers may be better able to care for the dying person.

2. The need to care and the need to be cared for sometimes conflict.

2. Those who sacrifice their own needs for care in order to care for others need to be encouraged to accept help for themselves. Some need to receive care before they can give care.

3. People vary in their coping abilities and personal resources. Moreover, competing priorities may hamper the amount and quality of care people are able to give.

3. Caregivers should not impose their own expectations on a family's ability to care. Caregivers may need to explore with the family what is reasonable for each person to provide.

4. The approach of death may disrupt the structure and functioning of the family.

4. Many families need counseling and support to prepare for the dying person's death and its consequences.

5. Families need to have information about a dying person's condition, although in cases of conflict his or her desire for confidentiality must be respected.

5. The dying person and caregiving team share the responsibility for informing the family about the person's condition, depending on his or her ability to participate. Whenever possible, the dying person and appropriate caregivers need to agree on the source and extent of information to be given to the family.

6. Families often need to be involved with the dying person in decision making.

6. Guided by the dying person's wishes, caregivers can be helpful in facilitating joint decision making.

7. Families have a right to know that their affairs will be shared only with those that have a need to know.

7. Confidentiality must be maintained at all times and its meaning taught to all caregivers.

8. Family members need to maintain self-esteem and self-respect.

8. Caregivers should show respect at all times. Caregivers do this by paying attention to family wishes, feelings, and concerns.

9. Sexual needs may continue up to the point of death.

9. Caregivers should acknowledge dying persons' and their partners' need to express their sexuality both verbally and physically, with easy access to privacy without embarrassment.

10. Families coping with terminal illness frequently have financial concerns.

10. Caregivers need to assure that families have access to informed advice and assistance on financial issues. These issues represent present or anticipated problems that may or may not be realistic.

11. Faced with death the family may imagine that changes will be greater than they are.

11. Caregivers can often allay fears with information and support.

12. Families have a need and a right to express grief for the multiple losses associated with illness, and for impending death.

12. Caregivers can help families by encouraging communication between families and the dying person about their shared losses, and encouraging the expression of grief.

Issues for Caregivers

ASSUMPTIONS

PRINCIPLES

1. Caregivers need education and experience in addressing the psychosocial needs of dying persons and their families.

1. A combination of specialized courses in death and dying, and clinical practicums in care of the terminally ill and their families, may help us to prepare caregivers to deal with the physical and psychosocial needs of dying persons.

2. Caregivers need to be aware of the dying person's and family's psychosocial frame of reference in acknowledging and coping with impending death.

2. Caregivers need to be sensitive to the dying person's and family's current willingness to acknowledge the reality of their situation. Caregivers must not impose their own expectation of how dying persons face death.

3. Caregivers bring their own values, attitudes, feelings, and fears into the dying person's setting.

3. Caregivers must recognize that they cannot take away all the pain experienced in the dying process. Caregivers need to be reassured that it is not a lack of professionalism to display and share emotions. Caregivers need to be aware of the way in which their coping strategies affect their communication of emotional involvement with the dying person and family.

4. Caregivers are exposed to repeated intense emotional experiences, loss, and confrontation with their own death in their work with dying persons.	4. Caregivers need to receive adequate support and opportunity to work through their own accumulated emotions. Caregivers working with dying persons need sound motivation, emotional maturity, versatility, tolerance, and a special ability to deal with loss.
5. Caregivers dealing with family groups sometimes experience conflicting needs and requests for information and confidentiality.	5. Caregivers need to be prepared to deal with complex family dynamics and to assist the family in resolving their own conflicts.
6. Caregivers may sometimes not communicate with each other about their own needs and feelings.	6. Caregivers need to be tolerant, caring, and nonjudgemental with each other in order to promote cooperation that will benefit the dying person's care.

To be effective, those who provide psychosocial services to terminally ill people and their families must develop a considerable sensitivity to the above issues. They must also learn to meet each dying patient as a unique individual with his or her own way of dying. Hospice can help patients grow emotionally and spiritually, but only if they wish to do so.

Some believe that dying patients should be offered an opportunity for growth by suggesting ways that they can develop themselves at the end of life. Others feel that the dying patient should determine the agenda and that encouraging the patient to deal with death and dying issues is intrusive.

There is some truth to both positions. It would be a mistake to be intrusive to patients and to expect them to be able to deal with their grief and unfinished interpersonal business before death. It would also be a mistake to passively avoid suggesting to them the same possibilities. Those facing death do not have prior experience on how best to die. The best one can do is offer them the possibility that there are opportunities to explore. If they show interest in dealing with feelings and relationships, hospice workers have permission to move forward. If they express discomfort, workers know to back off.

CASE ILLUSTRATION

Howard

Howard was the patriarch of a large family. At 78 years old, he had five children, 14 grandchildren, and eight great-grandchildren. His wife had died of a stroke 4 years earlier, and he was still feeling sad at her loss when he was diagnosed with Stage IV colon cancer. He opted for no oncology treatment and was admitted to hospice service.

As hospice staff got to know Howard, they began to learn more about his extraordinary life. He had traveled all over the world as a merchant seaman. He had become an engineer and had three patents registered. During World War II, he was parachuted behind enemy lines to sabotage enemy installations. He had been wealthy and had lost all his money on bad investments.

His family knew little of his exploits. One of his grandchildren was particularly interested in family history. The hospice social worker helped Howard to understand the importance of sharing his oral history with his family. Not only would their lives be enriched but his would be as well. Howard agreed to talk on videotape, beginning with what he could remember of his ancestors. He recounted the important details of his life. Finally, he shared his personal philosophy of life and thoughts on death and afterlife.

In the course of summarizing his life, he remembered some who had been major influences on him. He decided to write to two who were still living to thank them for their support and guidance. He also wrote a former business colleague who had been responsible for an important business failure. He forgave this old friend. As Howard's death approached, he thanked the hospice workers for helping him to reach closure on some important parts of his life.

TRUTH TELLING

Elisabeth Kübler-Ross once said that she used a rule of thumb about truth telling. She told her patients the truth three times and if after that they refused it she did not bring it up again. Clinical instincts can be helpful here. Timing is very important in any relationship. The first time you tell someone bad news, they often refuse to believe it. After they have had enough time to muster their more adaptive coping resources, they usually are able to hear it.

Robert Buckman (1992) gave some helpful guidance in *How to Break Bad News: A Guide for Health Care Professionals*. Buckman suggested a six-step protocol for breaking bad news. Step 1 is getting started by attending to the environment in which the bad news is given. Make sure there is enough privacy, be sure you are sitting down, and try to relax. Step 2 is to find out how much the patient knows. Ask open questions and look for factual knowledge as well as emotional content. Step 3 is to find out how much the patient wants to know. Again, it is best to ask open questions and try to discover at what level the patient wants to be informed. Questions like "Would you like to know the full details of what's wrong or just hear about the treatment plan?" are helpful. The fourth step is to share the information. Use of good communication skill is essential. Other suggestions include using plain English rather than "medspeak," give information in small chunks, use visual or written cues, and encourage questions. Step 5 is responding to the patient's feelings. A large number of responses are possible, including shock, denial, disbelief, fear, anxiety, anger, blame, guilt, hope, despair, depression, dependency, sadness, relief, joy, humor, bargaining, and a search for meaning. Finally in Step 6 is planning and follow-through. It is advisable to summarize what was said, to be sure all the options are explained, and to agree on the next steps. If there are no options, it is important to identify sources of support. It may still be possible to plan for the worst while hoping for the best.

Hospices are often in the difficult position of having to help people deal with the worst news they have ever received. Although patients are usually informed of their prognosis by a physician, it is the hospice worker who must help the patient and family to process this information. Once their shock wears off, there are numerous reactions. The significance of the patients' situation often has to be worked through over and over again.

In some respects, much of hospice care is helping people to face the truth. Patients and families have to be continuously reassessed to discern their readiness to digest more information. This becomes a delicate balancing act as the patients' conditions are continually changing.

When John was referred to hospice, he said he knew he was not supposed to recover but he preferred not to discuss it or think about it. The hospice team supported his request until 1 day a month later when he had an episode of incontinence. He laughed at himself as the home health aide changed his clothes and bathed him. He told his nurse that if he was going to keep from soiling himself he had better know more about his condition. This opened the door to talking about why he was losing bladder control and what other things might happen and how he could prepare. John discovered that he could cope better if he knew what to expect. His outlook changed, and he was less fearful and depressed.

SPIRITUALITY AND ACCEPTANCE OF DEATH

Are religious and spiritual needs synonymous? Hospice clinicians prefer to focus on patients' spiritual needs rather than limiting themselves to the religious. It is seen as a broader frame that encompasses both concerns with the rites, rituals, and rules of conventional religion and concerns with the individuals' desire to develop themselves spiritually.

Zerwekh (1993) described spirituality as the essence of personhood, the longing for meaning in existence, experience of God, experience of ultimate values, and trust in the transcendent. This is a broader frame that suits the situation of all dying patients whether they are religious, spiritual, or not. If one tries to understand patients' transcendent needs, one captures their religious, spiritual, philosophical, and existential concerns. By definition, any concern with why one is here or what happens after death concerns transcendence. People transcend their individual existences and are concerned with more than themselves.

Hospice chaplains and providers of care strive to help the patients get their transcendent issues in focus and to come to some resolution. The resolution can range from returning to good standing in their church or synagogue, to resolving their guilt over past transgressions, to feeling at peace with themselves and their notion of a universal power, to understanding what it is they needed to learn from their life, to acceptance or a sense that their life is complete and that they are ready to die.

Many patients and families are concerned about their religious beliefs as well as their spiritual lives. They may only know how to demonstrate their spirituality through religious expression. Hospices should always support the patient and family in the expression of their specific religious beliefs and practices and strive to learn those they are unfamiliar with.

Often, religious expression is influenced by cultural background. Each culture adapts religious expression to more comfortably fit cultural norms. Hospices are more effective when they understand these norms. Cultural beliefs and practices around death and dying are especially important for hospices to understand and support. For instance, hospice may help make it possible for an Islamic family to be able to wash and wrap the patient's body following death according to cultural and religious practice. The ability to carry out such perideath rituals can have a very positive impact on the bereavement process (see Irish, 1993, for more details on such practices).

Acceptance is more than just resignation toward death. Resignation is like learned helplessness. No matter what a person does, the illness progresses and one has to give in. There is no more point in fighting. Accepting death is an embracing of what comes next. It is a feeling of completeness with one's life without bitterness or regret. There is perhaps a sense of wonder about what lies ahead.

The following illustrates some of the difficult emotional challenges that face hospice providers and the potential to change a tragic situation into one in which there is some resolution.

CASE ILLUSTRATION

Janine

Janine was too young to die—only 37 years old with two small children, Josh (9) and Jackie (11). She had been fighting metastatic breast cancer for 4 years. Besides the tragedy of knowing she would not live to see her children grow up, there was a conflicted relationship with her ex-husband and a distant relationship with her parents. She had many friends and what she viewed as a good support system of other women.

Janine came to hospice after failing a round of chemotherapy. She was in need of help emotionally and physically, but she was not so sure about throwing in the towel. She could not say good-bye to her kids, and she felt very conflicted about her life. She was gradually getting weaker and spent most of her time in bed. Janine came into the hospice unit for pain control shortly after becoming a hospice patient. She could not get comfortable with increases in her morphine and was eventually put on a continuous subcutaneous infusion.

It became clear that increased doses of morphine were not affecting her pain. As we came to know Janine more, it became clear that she was agitated about who would care for her children when she was gone. She felt little trust for her husband, who had cheated on her, and she felt distant from her parents.

We explored with Janine what she could do to become more resolved about her children. We arranged for her parents to come and visit. They had not known how serious her illness had become. She invited her ex-husband to visit, but he would not show up when he said he would. Janine agreed that she would start a videotape of her life to leave for the children.

As her parents visited in the hospice unit, it became clear that the estrangement with her parents came from rebellion against them as a young adult. They had rejected her life-style and each had not forgiven the other for the angry things said. The conflict seemed almost trivial now that her life was near an end. They began to explore her life growing up to help with the video and to help her to put together a photo album. There was much sadness as they forgave each other and regret over the time they had lost.

Janine's pain was finally controlled, and she worked hard on the videotape project. She included special messages for her children. She left an oral history of her life, her philosophy, and her wishes. She went home to the care of her parents and friends. Arrangements were made for custody of the children to be given to her parents. Her ex-husband finally visited and asked for forgiveness for his behavior. He agreed to the custody arrangements and visited a few times although he was unable to stay long or to help with her care.

A week before she died, Janine finished her tape and family album. She spent as much time with Josh and Jackie as she could, and they helped with her care. She died peacefully in her bed with her parents, children, and friends around her. Two days later, they held a service that she had helped plan. Her children read some of her favorite poetry, and everyone celebrated her short but full life.

The dying face many intense emotional and spiritual concerns as death approaches. Grief is a central dynamic to the dying and especially to their families. In the next chapter, grief and bereavement are given more detailed attention.

RECOMMENDED READING

Becker, E. (1973). *The denial of death*. New York: Free Press.
Callanan, M., & Kelly, P. (1992). *Final gifts*. New York: Bantam Books.
Corless, I., Germino, B., & Pittman, M. (Eds.). (1994). *Dying, death and bereavement: Theoretical perspectives and other ways of knowing*. Boston: Jones & Bartlett.

Feifel, H. (1977). *New meanings of death*. New York: McGraw Hill.

Garfield, C. (Ed.). (1978) *Psychosocial care of the dying patient*. New York: McGraw Hill.

Kastenbaum, R. (1972). *The psychology of death*. New York: Springer.

Kübler-Ross, E. (1969). *On death and dying*. New York: Macmillan.

Levine, S. (1984). *Meetings at the edge*. New York: Doubleday.

Rosen, E. (1990). *Families facing death: Family dynamics of terminal illness*. Lexington, MA: Lexington Books.

Wass, H., & Neimeyer, R. (Eds.). (1995). *Dying: Facing the facts* (3rd ed.). Washington, DC: Taylor & Francis.

Weisman, A. D. (1972). *On dying and denying: A psychiatric study of terminality*. New York: Behavioral Publications.

Weenelson, P. (1996). *The art of dying: How to leave this world with dignity and grace, at peace with yourself and loved ones*. New York: St. Martin.

Grief and Bereavement

"A man's dying is more the survivor's affair than his own."

—Thomas Mann

The central psychological concern of patients and families facing death is reaction to loss. The patient faces the loss of everything, including health, occupation, body image, pleasures, significant relationships, and future. The family who will be left behind faces the loss of a loved one who is an integral part of a family system.

Hospices recognize that helping people deal with loss and grief is essential to providing good care. People do not begin to mourn a loss after the death, they begin as soon as the impending loss is acknowledged (Rando, 1986). This pre–death reaction is known as anticipatory grieving. It is generally accepted that some grieving is done before the loss; however, it is also held that the tasks of grieving cannot be completed before the actual loss.

There are a number of excellent texts on grief that the reader may wish to consult for a more in-depth exploration of the field (see end of chapter). This chapter focuses on how hospices provide bereavement services to hospice families as well as to the community at large. Special considerations for grieving children, prediction of bereavement risk, pathological grief identification, and cost effectiveness of bereavement support are also covered.

NEED FOR BEREAVEMENT SUPPORT

It would be fair to ask why hospices provide bereavement support in the first place. Isn't it the job of mental health agencies and churches to provide this service? To understand why hospices have emphasized a specialized bereavement support service, one needs to look at how society views the needs of the bereaved.

There is a tendency to minimize the impact of death on functioning. People are expected to be back to work or school and ready to function within a few days of the death. The average person thinks it should only take days or weeks to get over a death. The reality is that the first days or weeks are a period of shock. It is only after this time passes that a person is able to begin to deal with the loss.

There has been a breakdown in our sense of community. People have less time for friendship and often do not even know their neighbors. There is less social support available, and that support is critical to getting through a major loss. There are few cultural rituals to help people express grief. There is no commonly agreed-on etiquette for the public display of grief. People have fewer ties to organized religion and have reduced access to rituals and support from communities of faith. For those with such strong faith that they believed God would heal them, there may be a sense of failure or disappointment with God.

There is an assumption that clergy and mental health professionals are well trained in handling grief counseling. Few of these professionals receive any training in grief counseling or grief therapy. A few specialize in helping the bereaved, but the great majority have little knowledge or training in this area.

BEREAVEMENT FOLLOW-UP SERVICES

Hospices provide follow-up counseling, education, and support to families for a minimum of 1 year following the death. Hospice bereavement follow-up usually includes the following components:

1   Hospice clinical staff assigned to the case visit the family to say good-bye and to attend funeral or visitation.

2   A staff member or specially trained volunteer is assigned to contact the family at regular intervals in the year after the death.

3   Educational mailings are sent to families at regular intervals on aspects of grieving. Topics may include common reactions and feelings, journaling, poetry, self-esteem, next steps, and coping with holidays.

4   Hospice staff or volunteers are assigned to visit or call families at intervals determined by need. For those families without special needs, contact is usually after 1, 3, 6, 9, and 12 months. For families having trouble coping with grief, contact is more frequent or may require referral to a competent mental health professional with expertise in grief and loss.

5   Regular grief support groups are held, and all families are invited. These groups may include emotional support, educational components, or both. Some programs also include a social component.

The bereavement follow-up to a hospice family should be based on the needs identified. It may be helpful to see families as falling into one of four categories: those who refuse follow-up, those who need routine follow-up, those who need enhanced follow-up, and those whose mourning is complicated and who need professional intervention.

There are commonly a small number of families who ask for no further contact from hospice after the death. Usually it is because they are having some difficulty with their grief and prefer to use avoidance as a coping style. It may also be due to low self-esteem or tied to cultural expectations. Hospices respect this request and discontinue contact. However, it is recommended that at least one follow-up attempt be made after about 6 months to make sure that there has not been a change of heart. A significant number of these reluctant people find that their avoidance is ineffective and respond positively to follow-up. A hospice worker may hear, "I'm really glad you called; we're having more trouble dealing with this than I thought, and it would be good to talk about it."

The second group are those who welcome the contact from hospice and are coping well. These are the large majority of hospice families who have good support and coping resources. They do fine with a modest amount of follow-up. About 75% of families fall into this category.

The third group are those who need enhanced follow-up. These are the people who are having some difficulty with their grief and are having trouble coping. They may need or request more frequent contact from hospice. They are encouraged to come to the support groups and may require as much as weekly contact with hospice staff or volunteers.

The fourth group are those who have complicated or pathological grief. This may be manifested by severe depression, suicidal ideation, extreme difficulty in functioning, or unremitting distress. These family members are not responding to supportive intervention. They need to be helped to accept a referral for professional intervention. Hospice will have available or will have a referral relationship with mental health professionals in the community who are knowledgeable about treatment of grieving people. Often in this group, there is an underlying mental health problem that preexisted the loss.

COMMUNITY BEREAVEMENT SUPPORT

In a recent survey of U.S. hospices (Connor & Lattanzi-Licht, 1995), 88% reported that they provide bereavement services to the community at large, not just to families served by hospice. The most common community service was group counseling (94%), followed by phone support (82%), short-term counseling (72%), and educational mailings (72%). Other, less frequent types of support included an assigned volunteer (52%), long-term counseling (25%), expressive therapies (25%), and camp experiences (25%). Some hospices have even begun providing education and support through computer services and the Internet.

Often it is the families who were not served by hospice who use its bereavement services. Those served by hospice are usually more prepared for the death and may have fewer emotional complications afterward. Many communities view hospice as having expertise in handling grief and are turning to hospice programs for help in times of crisis.

Bereavement services for children tend to be easily accepted and valued by the community. Many hospices have developed special programs for schools and families with children. In the school system, hospices have led grief education programs, conducted debriefings after the deaths of students, and taught educators about grief and mourning. Some hospices use expressive therapists to work with children. These therapists use art, play, movement, storytelling, and other modalities to help children to express their grief.

Providing bereavement services for children and teens is especially important as a preventive measure. Children sometimes blame themselves for the death of a family member. They may either feel they caused the death or should have prevented it. Recently, a 5-year-old who had seen the movie "Twister" thought he caused a tornado because he had yelled out "Twister, twister" a while before a tornado destroyed the homes of most of his neighbors.

Teens have considerable fear of the public expression of grief for fear that it will alienate them from other, nongrieving peers. Both children and teens may be hesitant to bring up the subject of a loved one's death for fear that it might upset other family members. In some ways, providing services to children and teens is a way of reaching adults. It may be more acceptable for parents to seek help for their child than for themselves. In the process, they can receive help and education about their own grief.

Camps

Another popular community bereavement service are grief camps. This is a program where children go to a camp for a weekend or a number of days with hospice grief counselors and volunteers. There are entertaining and therapeutic activities planned. These might include craft programs designed to address grief such as making dream catchers to eliminate nightmares, worry dolls, and ornament decoration with objects from the deceased.

Activity programs at these camps might include physically challenging experiences such as ropes courses where group effort is necessary for success or mock survival situations. Art activity can help children express feelings and unresolved conflicts. Art or expressive therapists can help children understand the images or just reinforce the enjoyment of artistic creation.

Group rituals, where, for instance, participants may be asked to write down burdens that are then thrown into a fire, are common. Candles may be lit or other items may be sent floating down a river to symbolize loss. Trees may be decorated and then planted. Other group activities might include a memorial service, nondenominational religious observance, or family activity. The emphasis is on reducing the child's sense of isolation and feeling that he or she is the only one experiencing feelings of loss. It is also helpful for the child to deal with fears of losing other important people and guilt over perceived responsibility for the loss.

In most camps, the children come by themselves. There are some that both young and older children attend and others that are designed for teens or preteens only; some are designed for the whole family to attend. There is usually some type of follow-up activity after the camp, either through support groups or reunions. Participants describe the experience as a turning point where the loss finally was acknowledged or when the bad dreams finally went away.

Groups

Hospice grief support groups are usually open to the community at large. They are professionally facilitated self-help groups that are part of the common concern group movement that has flourished in the United States since the early 1970s. The structure and content of grief support groups varies. Some are open; others are closed. Open groups allow participants to come and go as they please. Closed groups usually require a commitment and are for a preset number of sessions. There are structured and unstructured group formats. Structured groups may offer a preset educational program with different topics for each session. Unstructured groups tend to follow the needs of the individuals who attend a particular session. Some offer a combination of topic for the session followed by an open support component.

Some hospices provide social occasions for the bereaved to attend. These are often potluck meals where widows and widowers come for good food, conversation, and sharing. As social support is an important factor in grief recovery, these occasions serve a therapeutic function. They have also been a springboard for other social contact and relationship building. Successful hospice socials have led to travel groups, bridge clubs, and sometimes to new marriages.

Counseling

Hospices vary in the amount of bereavement counseling offered. Most provide at least short-term counseling for anyone experiencing problems with grief. Some offer longer term counseling either using hospice staff or through arrangements with community therapists. This is usually on a sliding-scale fee basis. The objective of short-term counseling is to express grief and to help the person to progress through the normal tasks of mourning.

Worden (1991) has distinguished this from grief therapy, which aims to help someone whose grief is not progressing normally. Complicated grief may be due to preexisting psychological problems and may require a longer term therapy. Worden's conceptualization of grief work involves successfully completing four tasks. The first is accepting the reality of the loss. The second is feeling the pain of loss. The third is dealing with an environment without the deceased person, and the fourth is coming to a new relationship with the deceased that allows one to enter new relationships.

There has been discussion of the qualifications necessary to do grief counseling or therapy. The only well-recognized certification available is through the Association for Death Education and Counseling. Hospice staff who do grief counseling usually have a background in social work or pastoral care and receive on-the-job training. The great majority of family members' grief support needs can be met by using volunteers. Most hospices train volunteers to assist in providing support to the bereaved. In the United States, regular trained hospice volunteers will sometimes specialize in bereavement follow-up and be given some additional training.

In the United Kingdom, the Cruse Bereavement Care program was developed to provide a nationwide network of trained volunteers for the bereaved. This program provides free bereavement care for every grieving citizen in the country. Training for Cruse volunteers involves an initial 10-evening introduction followed by basic counseling training and a 60-hour supervised probation. The 6,000 Cruse volunteer counselors continue to be supervised as long as they stay in the program.

In the United Kingdom, specially trained individuals who receive more than 300 hours of training can be designated as counselors. These individuals are able to handle all the needs of the bereaved. In the United States, grief therapy is usually reserved for licensed mental health professionals with special expertise in grief work.

This dichotomy raises an interesting question about whether grief should be considered an abnormality. Most who work in hospice view grief as a fundamentally inherent part of the human experience. It is both a powerful human emotion and something that helps define who one is. The experience of loss can devastate but can also promote resiliency and strengthen the ties that bind people to others. Grief counseling may have emerged as a new social ritual to compensate for the loss of other forms of grief expression.

NORMAL VERSUS PATHOLOGICAL GRIEF

Current thinking in the mental health community is that bereavement can be a legitimate focus of treatment, but it does not constitute a mental disorder. Yet there are some whose reactions to loss are so overwhelming that they become unable to function.

Examples of pathological, complicated, or ineffective grief include the following: inhibited, delayed, prolonged, and exaggerated grief (Worden, 1991).

It is important to note that the range for what is normal grief is quite wide. Many times people seek counseling because they do not seem to be living up to society's unrealistic expectations that people simply pull up their bootstraps and get on with their life after a significant death. It is people's discomfort in having to acknowledge the griever's feelings that seems to push them to cut off the person's expression of grief.

A person with inhibited grief is unable to express feelings of grief. Some may have found ways of expressing their grief in nondistressing ways such as through creative expression; however, this type of person is usually troubled that he or she cannot express any feelings for the deceased. There may be an underlying fear that if any feeling is expressed the person will become overwhelmed.

In exaggerated grief, the person is flooded with grief and intense emotions and is unable to stop. Day and night, they feel pain and express painful emotion. Although it is helpful to express the pain of loss (Elisabeth Kübler-Ross [1969] called this emptying one's pool of pain), if it becomes a bottomless pit, help is needed. Sometimes this pain is not simply a result of the death but is related to other losses or traumas that have been unexpressed.

Delayed grief is found in those who after many months are unable to grieve and are distressed that they are unable to move on. The flip side of this is prolonged grief, where a person continues to grieve for years and cannot seem to stop.

In some cases, there is an obvious problem with a preexisting emotional problem that complicates grief. In other cases, though, there is no evidence of a mental disorder such as clinical depression or character disorder. Yet the person's ability to function is greatly impaired for a significant period.

Most theorists believe that major emotional expression is needed for grief to be resolved. Wortman and Silver (1989) questioned this need and claimed that some can resolve their grief without "feeling the pain." This may be a straw-dog argument as the expression of grief can take many forms and is as varied as human nature. Certainly one's cultural background has an enormous influence on the expression of mourning.

Can grief ever be resolved? Phyllis Silverman is a proponent of the life cycle model for understanding grief. This view is that grief is simply part of the normal life cycle. People grieve all their lives in one way or another. Grief helps to define who they are. Silverman objected to the medical model of grief as a wound that needs to be healed. One never finishes grieving and to expect people to do so may set them up for failure. This view is consistent with the report of many who say they will never completely get over their loss. If getting over the loss means the lack of any emotional connection to the deceased person, then most would prefer not to fully recover. This is not to say that it is not desirable to reach a place where grief does not preoccupy life.

Klass, Silverman, and Nickman (1996), in their recent book *Continuing Bonds*, explored the need for expanding the understanding of the grief process.

Most theorists have explained grief and mourning as a process aimed at cutting bonds with the deceased. Unhealthy grief is defined by how much the mourner continues to hold on to the dead person.

Yet experience with the bereaved helps one to understand that a continuing inner relationship with the deceased may not be unhealthy at all. Healthy resolution of grief enables people to maintain a continuing bond with the deceased that does not have to interfere with new relationships.

Bill Worden (1991) said that the most significant symptom that someone is having complicated grief is when the person is unable to be without an object of the deceased. He referred to this as a linking object. This object is usually a personal item that the bereaved has to have with them or know the location of at all times. The linking object signifies that the deceased remains the central emotional object in the life of the mourner. The grief of Queen Victoria is an example of someone whose life remained fixated on a lost relationship. She refused to stop mourning after the death of Prince Albert. His clothes were laid out daily and his place set at the table. She refused to accept the reality of his loss.

GRIEF AND DEPRESSION

One of the most difficult clinical distinctions is between grief and depression. They have many of the same characteristics, but the most distinguishing differences are that in depression there is a pervasive disturbance of self-esteem, hopelessness, psychomotor retardation, or suicidal gestures that greatly affect social and occupational functioning (Jacobs & Leiberman, 1987). There are more vegetative signs and symptoms in depression, which are less typical of an acute stress reaction. In grief the pain of loss is recognized, whereas in depression it is unrecognized and denied. Anger is more easily expressed in grief than in depression. Grieving people are more preoccupied with the deceased, whereas depressed people are more focused on themselves. Grievers usually respond well to support, whereas depressed people do not and will tend to drive others away.

Another difficult grief reaction is feeling excessive guilt. Probably most mourners experience some guilt as they go over the events of the death, seeking reassurance that all was done that could be done. Illegitimate guilt may be a defense against helplessness. It is easier to take responsibility for the event than to accept the randomness of the world and not feel in control. Exploring the legitimacy of the guilt may help get at underlying assumptions. When guilt is legitimate, it can be channeled into constructive activity and, it is hoped, changes into forgiveness and feelings of regret.

One way to understand and work with grief is to focus on the stories of the bereaved. The story of the events leading up to, during, and right after the death are of major significance to the bereaved. How the narrative evolves and is interpreted has a significant impact on the course of bereavement. Hospice families are often told that it is most helpful to tell their story, and they do it over and over again.

Stroebe and Shut (1995) have proposed a new model for understanding grief in adult life. They proposed a dual-process model for grief that accounts for the vacillation in the emotional responses seen in the bereaved. Most people have periods after a major loss where they avoid the emotional reactions characteristic of grief. There are many practical details that must be attended to after a death. These reality-based concerns allow a break from the more intense emotional work of grief.

Everyday life experience oscillates between loss-oriented activities such as grief work, intrusive emotional reactions, untying bonds, and restorative activities such as attending to life changes, doing new things, distraction from grief, and denial or avoidance of grief (Stroebe & Shut, 1995). In this model, there are no stages or phases of grief, just a continuing oscillation. Difficulty occurs when the person cannot move back and forth and stays stuck either in loss or in the restorative activities.

Most researchers have agreed that red flags for complicated grief include

- when a person is thinking about hurting him- or herself
- when a person feels constantly depressed and unable to find a glimmer of hope
- when a person refuses to seek medical help for health problems
- when a person starts drinking more or taking illegal drugs to soothe grief
- when a person feels constantly guilty or angry at the deceased
- when a person refuses to talk about the deceased or has difficulty expressing any emotions

In spite of the many helpful theories about and models of grief, a truly integrated universal theory of bereavement is still lacking. Researchers tend to define unhealthy grief as any behaviors that do not fit their simplistic models of how people ought to grieve.

RISK FOR POOR OUTCOME

Much of the bereavement literature concerns identification of those individuals who are at risk for poor outcome in their grief. Poor outcome usually means development of emotional disorders, suicide, or health deterioration. There is disagreement in the literature as to whether grief can cause illness or death. In Osterweis, Solomon, and Green's (1984) *Bereavement: Reactions, Consequences, and Care,* the risk literature is reviewed and found to lack sufficient proof for having a causal relationship with morbidity and mortality. The cause is often attributed to grief after the fact owing to proximity.

Stroebe and Stroebe (1987) later reviewed the field in *Bereavement and Health* and came to a different view. They found evidence to support a strong relationship between widowhood and poor health outcomes. In their review of the risk literature, they showed that the only well-established risk factors are male gender, young age, and lack of forewarning. There is also quite a bit of evidence for perceived lack of social support.

The other factors studied, including (a) social class, (b) race and ethnicity, (c) religiosity, (d) personality, and (e) prior health history, did not have enough evidence to be established as risk factors at this time.

Catherine Sanders (1993) summarized findings on risk factors in bereavement outcome and concluded that the following factors can be seriously debilitating:

- ambivalence and dependency
- parental bereavement
- health before bereavement
- concurrent crises
- perceived lack of social support
- age and gender (young age, male sex)
- reduced material resources

Recent articles (Avis, Brambilla, Vass, & McKinlay, 1991; Barry & Fleming, 1988; Wolinsky & Johnson, 1992) have continued this debate about causality. One generally accepted observation is that bereaved people tend to have greater utilization of the health care system. This may be due to increased illness or to mental health reasons. After the death of a spouse, it is natural for a widowed person to seek support through accepted venues. If one is distressed, it is acceptable to go to the doctor. It may also be that taking care of one's ailments is put on hold in the period preceding a spouse's death and that these accumulated complaints are dealt with afterward.

COST EFFECTIVENESS OF BEREAVEMENT FOLLOW-UP

A recent study by Connor (1996a) found that an association existed between being a widowed person who received bereavement follow-up through hospice and a decrease in the use of health care resources in the year following the death. A total of 354 widowed persons were studied over a 2-year period. In this time-series designed study, there were three groups. The control group of 111 bereaved spouses received no follow-up. A limited-intervention group of 128 received a minimal follow-up consisting of four components. The third, extensive-intervention group of 115 received hospice services and a more extensive follow-up consisting of seven components.

Use of inpatient and outpatient health care services in the year before and year after the spouses' death was analyzed. Data on all scheduled outpatient services, both physician and nonphysician, were compiled. Data on all inpatient days were also collected for each participant. Clinic data for each group were analyzed by using a T test for independent means to determine if the difference scores from the year before the death to the year after the death were significant. Results indicated that there was no significant difference between the no-intervention and limited-intervention groups. There was, however, a significant difference between the extensive-intervention (hospice) group and the no-intervention group ($p < .001$). This reduction amounted to an average of two clinic visits per participant.

More notable results were found in the inpatient data. Again, the limited-intervention group had reduction in hospital use compared with the no-intervention group (345 days vs. 166 days), but the difference was not significant. For the hospice group, however, there was a significant difference between the no-intervention group (345 days vs. 49 days, $p < .0001$) This difference amounted to an average of about 3 hospital days per participant.

Hospice bereavement counseling and follow-up may be associated with reduced use of health care services. Spouses who were involved with the care of their loved one before the death and received support before, during, and after the death seemed to have fewer health complaints.

CURRENT ISSUES IN BEREAVEMENT

The *Handbook of Bereavement* (Stroebe, Stroebe, & Hansson, 1993) offers a thorough summary of some of the emerging themes, results, and controversies in the bereavement field.

Grief is not a universal process with typical symptoms. There are a wide range of individual and cultural differences in the way people grieve. What is normal in one culture may be quite abberrant in another. Adjustment to bereavement is a multifactorial process involving far more than emotional responses. Research is needed to look more at the full range of behavioral and cognitive reactions as well.

Stage theories may help one understand in a general way how people form attachments (Bowlby, 1980/1981) or respond to stress (Horowitz, 1986), but they do not help one to understand a particular individual. Bereavement may not always result in distress but can usually be expected rather than being inevitable. Researchers do not yet understand the universality of grief, though grief-like responses have been found in very diverse societies and across species. More in-depth research is needed on the differing patterns of loss found in different cultures.

The duration of grief and recovery continues to be a controversial topic. Most agree that the majority of bereaved persons cease to grieve intensely after 1 or 2 years. However, a return to baseline does not equal recovery. Some forms of grieving may never end, and when there has been a strong attachment, emotional involvement with the deceased is likely to continue throughout life.

Are there differences in grief reactions following different types of loss? Is the loss of a limb or a farm as bad as the loss of a life partner? These questions remain hard to reconcile. Different types of loss may require special needs be attended to for maximum benefit.

Although there is evidence for an excess mortality rate among bereaved person, there is still a great deal researchers need to know about the impact of bereavement on health. Also, although some factors may predispose someone to be more vulnerable to poor outcome in bereavement, there continues to be controversy over which factors they are and whether they are unique to bereavement or are associated with poor health in the population at large.

An examination of effective versus ineffective coping is a central research concern. Is suppression of memories an effective coping strategy or is it essential to develop a tolerance for memories of the deceased?

Finally, research on the efficacy of bereavement support and intervention has pointed toward the usefulness of providing assistance to bereaved persons. However, much more work is needed to identify who benefits most from which interventions. With the breakdown in social support networks, more formal support services are needed to compensate. As can be seen from the above, the bereavement field is still in need of a great deal of study.

Most would agree that how people grieve is affected a great deal by their life experiences with loss. These experiences can set a pattern for how people deal with loss throughout the life span. The following two cases are examples of how complicated grief can emerge and be dealt with.

CASE ILLUSTRATIONS

Trudy

Trudy was a 63-year-old widow whose husband had died of pancreatic cancer as a hospice patient. She was a social worker who was still working. She was an excellent caregiver who seemed to be coping well with her grief. After Fred's death in the hospice unit, she seemed numb for a month or so. The hospice volunteer who stayed in contact with her said she was not expressing any emotion and seemed to be stuck in her grief after several months.

Trudy came for individual counseling to assist her in moving through the grief process. She knew that Fred was dead, but she did not feel particularly sad and this bothered her. She felt mostly alone and a little overwhelmed. She missed Fred and at times had the feeling that he was still there. She thought she heard or saw him in brief glimpses.

In the course of therapy, Trudy showed a tendency to become dependent on me as her therapist and to be needy. She would become anxious if unable to make her appointment. As she recounted her life history, she focused a lot on her father. He was larger than life, and his death 20 years ago had been a great blow to her. As with Fred, she had been unable to grieve for him after he died.

As we explored the relationship with her father for clues to her current limitation, troubling memories began to come to light. She remembered that some 50 years ago her father had molested her as a teenager. The experience had devastated her. She felt like an object rather than a person. She relived the experience as if it were yesterday.

Fred had been the savior who had taken her away, and now that he was gone she felt too vulnerable. She felt both anger and sadness about her relationship with her father. Many thoughts and feelings had to be expressed about this basic violation of trust before she could begin to express long-lost feelings of grief for her father and for the father he would never be.

Finally, she was able to express her pain at the loss of her husband. He had been a good husband and father, but she had always kept a part of herself away from him for fear that he would break her trust, too. Now that he was gone, she also grieved for the loss of the relationship she could not have with him because of her long-buried secret.

As these issues and feelings came to light, her ability to function as an independent person improved. She learned to take care of all the things Fred had done and to keep herself focused at work. As she terminated therapy, she was getting involved in many new outside activities that she had not had the courage to do before.

Margaret

Margaret was a 60-year-old widow whose husband had died 18 months earlier. She was referred by the mental health department of our medical center due to unremitting grief. Her husband had died suddenly of a heart attack. In our first session, she was convinced that nothing would help. She knew he was dead, and she was caught up in the intense pain of her grief.

Margaret had been very dependent on her husband for everything. He had made all decisions for her, and she had relied on him in a childlike manner. Her own father had died in an accident when she was 14. She felt completely alone and bereft in the world. She wanted someone to tell her that she would recover and it would be all right. In spite of this wish, she was easily angered and rejected all attempts at reassurance from friends whom she had driven away through her continuous expression of painful grief.

She was isolated and complained of depressive symptoms. Her sleep was poor, along with her appetite. She enjoyed nothing and had difficulty thinking clearly. She had been taking an antidepressant but with little improvement.

Margaret had a long-standing history of emotional problems that preceded her bereavement. Before much progress could be made, a stable therapeutic relationship was needed. She had not developed emotionally, and it seemed like she was behaving much like a 14-year-old whose emotional outbursts could not be controlled.

After some trust was developed, we explored what had happened following the accidental death of her father. There had been a period of intense emotional reaction followed by a complete absence of grief. During her remaining teen years, she became withdrawn and could not express emotion except for occasional angry outbursts. She became very dependent on her mother. She married after high school and went from her mother's home to her husband's without ever having lived on her own.

Margaret came to see that her father's death had taken away what sense of basic trust she had had. Her response was to contain her emotions (particularly her anger at her father for leaving her) as best she could and to be dependent on others. When her husband died, it reactivated the conflicts she had never resolved as an adolescent. Over a course of therapy, she had to learn how to gain a sense of safety, control, connection, and identity, the building blocks of personhood that had not been gained following the death of her father.

I now turn from the more clinical aspects of hospice care to the larger issues of hospice's role within a community. The next chapter looks at how hospices have come to be the focal point in many communities for helping society to move toward a healthier understanding of death, dying, and bereavement.

RECOMMENDED READING

Bowlby, J. (1980a). *Attachment and loss: Attachment*. New York: Basic Books.

Bowlby, J. (1980b). *Attachment and loss: Separation—Anxiety and anger*. New York: Basic Books.

Cook, A., & Dworkin, D. S. (1992). *Helping the bereaved: Therapeutic interventions for children, adolescents and adults*. New York: Basic Books.

Dershimer, R. (1990). *Counseling the bereaved*. New York: Pergamon Press.

Grollman, E. (Ed.). (1980). *What helped me when my loved one died*. Boston: Beacon Press.

Klass, D., Silverman, P., & Nickman, S. (Eds.). (1996). *Continuing bonds: New understandings of grief*. Washington, DC: Taylor & Francis.

Lattanzi-Licht, M., Kirschling, J. M., & Fleming, S. (Eds.). (1989). *Bereavement care: A new look at hospice and community based services*. New York: Hayworth Press.

Osterweis, M., Solomon, F., & Green, M. (Eds.). (1984). *Bereavement: Reactions, consequences, and care*. Washington, DC: National Academy Press.

Parkes, C. M. (1987). *Bereavement: Studies of grief in adult life* (2nd ed.). New York: International Universities Press.

Parkes, C. M., & Weiss, R. (1983). *Recovery from bereavement*. New York: Basic Books.

Rando, T. (1984). *Grief, dying and death: Clinical interventions for caregivers*. Champaign, IL: Research Press.

Rando, T. (1984). *Loss and anticipatory grief*. Lexington, MA: Lexington Books.

Rando, T. (1993). *Treatment of complicated mourning*. Champaign, IL: Research Press.

Raphael, B. (1983). *The anatomy of bereavement*. New York: Basic Books.

Silverman, P. (1986). *Widow to widow*. New York: Springer.

Stroebe, W., & Stroebe, M. (1987). *Bereavement and health*. New York: Cambridge University Press.

Stroebe, M. S., Stroebe, W., & Hansson, R. O. (1993). *Handbook of bereavement: Theory, research, and intervention*. New York: Cambridge University Press.

Tatelbaum, J. (1980). *The courage to grieve*. New York: Lippencott & Crowell.

Worden, W. J. (1991). *Grief counseling and grief therapy: A handbook for the mental health practitioner* (2nd ed.). New York: Springer.

Community Education

HOSPICE'S ROLE IN EDUCATING THE COMMUNITY

Community-based hospices have made it a part of their mission to educate communities about hospice care and issues around death and dying. Hospice has always been in part a consumer movement. As consumers of health care, the public has learned to become wary of the promises of modern medicine.

Medicine promises to remedy all ills and views death as an enemy to be defeated. People want to believe physicians when they say there is much that can be done to cure the disease. They want to believe surgeons when they say they got all the cancer. They want to believe that they will be one of the 5% who will respond to the new treatment. Elderly people tend to be more careful when facing medical decisions. They have seen friends and family who died alone and in pain in the hospital. They know of the disappointment after false hope has been dashed.

The recent SUPPORT Investigators (1995) study demonstrated that death in the U.S. health care system is still characterized by ignorance of patients' treatment wishes. As previously mentioned, this 2-year prospective observational study was an attempt to improve end-of-life decision making and to reduce the frequency of mechanically supported, painful, and prolonged dying.

A total of 4,301 patients participated in this two-phase study at five teaching hospitals in the United States. The first phase involved studying how patients died in the hospital and documented shortcomings in communication and the frequency of aggressive treatment administered. Findings from Phase 1 included that only 47% of physicians knew when their patients preferred to avoid CPR, 46% of physicians knew of do-not-resuscitate (DNR) orders that were written within 2 days of death, 38% of patients who died spent at least 10 days in an intensive care unit, and for 50% of conscious patients who died in the hospital, family members reported moderate to severe unrelieved pain at least half the time.

Even more troubling were findings from Phase 2 of the study. In an effort to improve the care of hospitalized dying patients, SUPPORT Investigators (1995) assigned specially trained nurse advocates to help make patients' treatment wishes known. They also developed a sophisticated algorithm that helped predict the probability of a patient's death within a time span (Lynn, Tino, & Harell, 1995). Results of these prognostic reports were provided to physicians to help them more accurately determine which patients were nearing death.

During Phase 2 of the SUPPORT Investigators (1995) study, intervention patients experienced no improvement in patient–physician communication. Five areas were targeted to show positive outcomes: discussion of CPR preferences, timing of DNR orders, physician knowledge of CPR preferences, number of days spent in the intensive care unit, and level of reported pain. The intervention also did not reduce use of hospital resources.

These findings demonstrate what many in the hospice field already knew, that there is a great deal of room for improvement in the care of dying patients in the health care system. They also show that a concerted well-orchestrated interdisciplinary effort is needed to deal with the complex and highly emotional issues surrounding dying.

The SUPPORT Investigators (1995) underestimated the difficulty of appropriately caring for the dying when they designed the study. They thought that all that would be needed was a little education for the patients, families, and physicians, and a major change would occur. They underestimated the tenacity of physicians in continuing to care for patients the way they always have. They did not see that for a major change to occur in the way patients were cared for, a multidisciplinary educational effort was needed.

Hospices know that they have a message that everyone needs to hear but that few wish to hear. In spite of 20 years of grass-roots activity and concerted efforts at educating the public, most people still do not seem to have a clue as to what hospice does. There is usually a vague idea that it has to do with care of the dying, but few facts are known. A common misconception in the United States is that hospice is a place where people go to die. In the United Kingdom, this is closer to the truth.

Unless someone in your family or a close friend has used the services of hospice it's unlikely that you will know much about it. When someone needs the services of hospice, he or she is usually amazed at the services available. Yet even those who have direct experience receiving hospice care tend not to discuss it too often and relegate it along with the painful memories of the death.

In essence, the hospice movement reminds people that death is a natural part of life and that they must take that knowledge into account whenever they make a treatment decision. How one dies is just as important as how long one lives.

AVOIDANCE

So why after two decades of care for a large segment of the population is hospice and palliative care still so little known? In spite of the culture's and media's fascination with unnatural death, people avoid anything having to do with natural death. They prefer to ignore anything that reminds them that they will have to face their own deaths someday.

The denial that is pervasive in society inhibits people from choosing to face the facts surrounding death and dying. Few people seek out an opportunity to become educated about death, grief, and loss. When they are exposed to the reality of death, they usually tend to put it out of mind as quickly as possible. Perhaps it is like staring at the sun: A person cannot do so for long.

In annual in-services on hospice care given to hospital staff, the people attending seem to retain little from one year to the next. They ask what exactly it is that hospice does. Newsletters are sent out, educational mailings are done, articles in the newspapers are printed, and talks are given to all sorts of community groups, all to little avail. If one asked the average person what hospice is they would be apt to say "I'm not sure."

Hospices have tried various strategies to make their message less difficult to hear. They have come up with various euphemisms for death. Instead of describing clients as *terminally ill,* they are now described as having a life-threatening illness or a life-limiting illness. Even the word *hospice* is a word with little prior connection to death. However, any word chosen will eventually become tainted by association with the reality of the work that is done. There is considerable discussion in the field about dropping the word *hospice* in favor of *palliative care.* This may reflect that hospice has become too identified with a narrowly defined set of services and structures. Whatever name is used to describe an effort to care for the dying will be difficult for people to embrace.

TRAUMA RESPONSE

Some hospice programs have begun to expand their bereavement outreach programs to include services for victims of traumatic death. The whole field of trauma research and response has mushroomed in recent years. Large-scale disasters such as the Oklahoma City bombing have propelled the needs of victims into the public's eye. On the local level, there are numerous tragic events that leave victims in their wake. Hospices are a natural resource for providing ongoing support to victims.

The field of trauma response is generally divided into two major groups, the victim assistance organizations (such as the National Organization for Victim Assistance) and the emergency responder groups. Many states in the United States now have posttrauma response teams that can be readily mobilized to respond to either a major disaster or a local emergency.

These response groups are usually able to provide short-term services such as debriefing victims or emergency responders, defusing participants in an ongoing traumatic scene, or doing school intervention. Their intervention is in the period immediately after the crisis and is aimed at prevention of later posttraumatic stress responses in participants. Except for unusual and large-scale disasters, there is little or no ongoing service.

Hospices can be part of the continuum of posttrauma response by offering a variety of services. They can assist in the initial debriefing of victims by participating in or offering to provide posttrauma response services. Some are working with local law enforcement to help them in responding to traumatic death by, for instance, having specially trained staff or volunteers who can accompany officers who must inform family of a traumatic death.

Hospice can add to the community response by providing ongoing services. Support groups or individual counseling can be offered to victims who continue to need to express reactions to the loss. Social support and social work assistance can be provided to the bereaved to help them adjust to life without the deceased. Chaplains can help victims cope with their anger at God. For those who are suffering more severe impairment, hospice can serve as a bridge for referral to mental health.

VOLUNTEER TRAINING

Hospices have always relied on volunteers to help in caring for patients. All hospice volunteers must go through an extensive training program before assisting in care. They receive training in basics such as psychological reactions to death and dying, grief and loss, personal death awareness, confidentiality, documentation, the interdisciplinary team, and so forth.

Hospice volunteer training programs act as a community education service. Many of the people who attend these programs do not end up as volunteers. They come to learn about hospice or to help them deal with their own death anxiety.

As many as half of those who attend self-select themselves out. A few are eased out by the volunteer trainers if there are apparent emotional problems or agendas for volunteering that are inconsistent with hospice. If someone has had a recent bereavement, wishes to convert others to a faith before dying, or is there to meet their own needs more than those of the patient and family, they are not appropriate for work in hospice.

HOSPICE IN THE SCHOOL SYSTEM

Schools have been quite receptive to education from hospice programs. Requests for presentations on subjects such as death and dying, loss and grief, trauma, advanced directives, and so forth have proven hospice's value to the educational community.

Elementary and secondary educators are aware that there is very little opportunity to teach children about death in the current school curriculum. Children are very inquisitive about end-of-life issues, and teachers have very little experience in how to discuss the topic. Schools reflect society, which still has difficulty acknowledging that death is a part of life. Bringing in outside experts on the topic helps children learn to respond to death in healthier ways and relieves teachers who are sometimes fearful of mishandling the topic.

Where hospices have shown their expertise and given help to schools, schools have responded by giving hospices increased access and in some cases funding for their outreach activity. A typical scenario might include coming as a guest speaker for students, followed by doing training for school personnel, followed by being asked to respond to help groups of students following the death of a student, to giving memorial services, to doing ongoing groups and classes for students or teachers.

As schools learn that hospices can be trusted to work within the education system, there are sometimes funds available to support outside consultation and education. These funds can be requested by hospice for services performed. Schools can also be prime referral sources for other support services for students such as grief camps, groups, or other activities put on by hospices.

Community colleges can also be forums for community education on hospice topics. Some hospices have banded together to conduct a course on hospice for the community.

There is also a growing interest in offering courses on death and dying as part of graduate and undergraduate curriculums. Most psychology programs have an elective course on death and dying. Several universities also offer a degree program in thanatology, the study of death and dying.

EDUCATIONAL ORGANIZATIONS

The Association for Death Education and Counseling is a national organization that provides certification programs for death educators and counselors who specialize in working with the dying and bereaved. The association holds annual conferences and ongoing training programs for members to distinguish them as qualified to teach and counsel.

The NHO is the largest organization representing the interests of hospices in the United States. Rather than being a trade organization, it is a nonprofit corporation that seeks to further care for the dying in the United States. NHO's primary activity is to provide education to hospices and related organizations and individuals. It conducts an annual meeting, an annual management conference, and several specialty conferences throughout the United States.

NHO coordinates a council of hospice professionals made up of 14 sections representing different disciplines and activities within hospices. There are sections for CEOs and executive directors, administrators, nurses, social workers, spiritual caregivers, bereavement professionals, allied therapists, nursing assistants, public relations and development specialists, funeral directors, physicians, pharmacists, social workers, volunteers, and researchers, academics, and educators. Each section has regular meetings and a newsletter to share activities and to promote networking within respective hospice disciplines.

Each state has a hospice association that promotes hospice care at the state level. NHO has a Council of States that is made up of the leadership of the state associations. The council has its own newsletter and attempts to coordinate education on a regional level for hospice programs. Education for hospice professionals is primarily done at the state and regional levels.

The National Hospice Foundation is affiliated with NHO. It is a foundation whose purpose is to promote education and research in hospice care. The foundation has sponsored a number of important activities, including physician education teleconferences and a touring photographic exhibit on hospice care.

The Hospice Association of America is the second national organization focused on promotion of hospice care. The Hospice Association of America is a part of the National Association for Home Care. This association is the national trade organization that represents the home health industry in the United States. In recent years, it has been trying to broaden its scope to include all health care activities that occur in the home. It is reaching out to the providers of paraprofessional services in the home, durable medical equipment providers, home infusion and mobile health service providers. Many home health agencies that are members of the National Association for Home Care also provide hospice services, and the association is attempting to expand to be a major voice for hospice through the Hospice Association of America. Hospice educational programs are conducted as part of the National Association for Home Care's national and regional educational programs.

The National Prison Hospice Association promotes hospice care for terminally ill inmates and those facing the prospect of dying in prison in the United States. The goal of this association is to support and assist corrections professionals and outside groups in their continuing efforts to develop patient care procedures and management programs in the prison systems.

The Canadian organization that represent the interests of palliative and hospice care providers north of the U.S. border is the Canadian Palliative Care Association. Every 2 years, an international conference on palliative care is held in Montreal, Quebec, Canada. Dr. Balfour Mount (a pioneer palliative care physician) founded the conference, which is focused on expanding clinical knowledge of palliative care.

The European Association for Palliative Care has been formed to assist in the development of palliative care services throughout Europe. Conferences are organized, technical assistance is given, and the *European Journal of Palliative Care* is published for members and others.

EDUCATING THE MEDICAL COMMUNITY

One of the hospice movement's original goals was to improve care of the dying in the health care system to such an extent that hospices would not need to exist. After more than 20 years, it appears that hospice is a long way from achieving that goal. As shown in the SUPPORT Investigators (1995) study, those dying in the health care system are still too often alone, in pain, and overtreated.

So how are health care professionals to be taught not only the skills of palliative care but the judgment and values that are necessary when caring for those who are incurably ill? Medicine and nursing teach that the preservation of life is paramount. The pursuit of this ideal is well intentioned but becomes perverted when it seeks to prolong life at any cost to the person.

Changing physician attitudes must be done as early as possible. At present, the most exposure the usual medical student gets to death and dying is one lecture during the course of a 4-year education. There are some medical schools and residency programs that include opportunities to learn about palliative care, but these are rare.

The Agency for Health Care Policy and Research (1994) recently published guidelines for treating pain. One of its findings was that physicians received little training in pain management. In an effort to redress this lack, the National Institutes of Health recommended that funds be allocated to develop model training programs in hospice and palliative care for physicians. Proposals were received from hospices, medical schools, and residency training programs. A number of programs were funded in 1995 to develop curriculums and physician–resident training models, including the American Academy of Hospice and Palliative Medicine; Hospice of the Florida Suncoast; the West Coast Palliative Care Center at the University of California, Davis; and Dartmouth.

This effort is a small step in the right direction. It is only a small first attempt. What is needed is support from those who control decisions about medical school curriculum. Medicine has grown so complex that there is hardly any room available in the 4-year curriculum for new content. Yet controlling pain and caring for people who are incurably ill are a significant part of a physician's duties in practice.

Another approach is to focus on developing specialty training for those physicians and health care professionals who are interested in care of the dying. In the United Kingdom, palliative medicine is a recognized subspecialty. There are posts established, and the need for physicians with this specialty has been analyzed so that an adequate number are being trained. There is also a diploma program for physicians of any specialty to obtain training in palliative medicine while remaining in practice. Canada has also developed a curriculum for physician training. The United States remains behind in the recognition of palliative care and palliative medicine.

The American Academy of Hospice and Palliative Medicine is an association of physicians working in hospice and palliative care. The Adacemy holds a high-level annual clinical workshop and has recently established a certification exam for physicians wishing to be recognized for experience in palliative medicine.

In nursing, there are some efforts to provide specialized training in hospice and palliative care. The Hospice Nurses Association now offers a certification program for hospice nurses. A nurse must take and pass a national exam to become a certified hospice nurse. Too often, nurses are hired to work in hospices and after a brief orientation are expected to be able to function as hospice nurses. Given the burgeoning literature on palliative care and the level of responsibility given to hospice nurses, it is reasonable to expect hospice nurses to receive considerable training before being asked to manage the care of a dying patient.

Recently, social work standards were written for social workers who work in hospices (NHO, 1994b). These standards specify the training and experience needed for a hospice social worker.

SUPPORT GROUPS

Many hospices formed out of support groups for cancer patients and those grieving a loss. These common concern groups emerged in the 1970s as part of the self-help movement (Alcoholics Anonymous, Parents Without Partners, Widow to Widow Program, Compassionate Friends, etc.). People need to feel they have some sense of control over their problems. They need information and learn best from others who have faced the same problems that they are facing.

Today, support groups remain an important part of a hospice's scope of services. Hospices facilitate groups for a large variety of populations. In addition to cancer support, there are groups for people living with AIDS, caregiver support groups, and groups for specific disease populations such as breast cancer, laryngectomy, women's cancer issues, motor neuron disease, and so forth. In addition to general grief support groups, there are groups for survivors of suicide, murder victims, AIDS, death of children, and so forth.

Groups range in style and content. Some are open and others are closed after the first few sessions. Some are highly structured, and others vary depending on the needs of the participants attending a given session. Most include an education component. Some are nearly all educational, whereas others are nearly all support focused. Hospices often hold open sessions for the community to learn more about services. These are usually free sessions offering education to the public on topics such as preparing for death, making an advanced directive, how to care for an ill relative, and the like. These sessions offer the public an opportunity to learn more about hospice services, to value what hospices have to offer, and to overcome misconceptions about hospice care.

It is clear that for the hospice movement to succeed, hospice must become an everyday word for the public. This will not occur as long as hospice is seen as an anomaly in the health care system that is available only to a few. Hospices must speak out loudly in the current debate over the right to die. They must make their presence known and be willing to reach out to all dying patients who face the end of life.

RECOMMENDED READING

Corless, I., Germino, B., & Pittman, M. (Eds.). (1995). *A challenge for living: Dying, death and bereavement*. Boston: Jones and Bartlett.

Corr, C., Nabe, C., & Corr, D. (1994). *Death and dying, life and living*. Pacific Grove, California: Brooks/Cole.

DeSpelder, L., & Strickland, A. (1992). *The last dance: Encountering death and dying* (3rd ed.). Mountain View, CA: Mayfield.

Kastenbaum, R., & Kastenbaum, B. (Eds.). (1989). *Encyclopedia of death*. Phoenix, AZ: Oryx Press.

Wass, H., & Neimeyer, R. (Eds.). (1995). *Dying: Facing the facts* (3rd ed.). Washington, DC: Taylor & Francis.

Part Two

Pitfalls

In this section, the reader will find a discussion of the unique difficulties associated with operating a hospice program. These four chapters look at how hospice care is organized and financed in the United States and how managed care is affecting the delivery of hospice care. Also included is information on how the right-to-die movement is affecting hospice and how our society's difficulty with death has limited hospice.

Chapter Seven

The Realities of Hospice Management

"There go my people. I must find out where they are going so I can lead them."

—Alexandre Ledru-Rollin

WE DON'T MAKE WIDGETS

Providing leadership in a hospice program is one of the most challenging roles anywhere. A hospice must be run as a business and at the same time ought to function as a venue for the noble expression of humanity. This is not suggested out of misty-eyed sentimentality.

Where hospices may have lost their souls, it is because the demands of the business have overshadowed the essential vision of hospice: a community of people dedicated to the relief of suffering, who help make possible opportunities for growth at the end of life.

There is an ongoing tension between the demands of business survival and the need to preserve what is important and unique about hospice. There are also some who never understood hospice's mission in the first place and simply look on it as a product line, marketing device, or cost-effective way of caring for some of the more expensive patients in the health care system.

In most businesses, the essential purpose of the group's activity is simple. The corporation exists for self-preservation through the creation of profits. Profits are made if the product or service produced can be sold for more than it costs to produce. The greater the demand for the product or service, the larger the business.

Many businesses now realize that organizational self-preservation, profits, and growth can be enhanced by reframing the company as it exists for the purpose of delivering quality goods or services. The total quality management movement in manufacturing is spreading to the service industries. The more successful companies see themselves as existing for the purpose of providing a superior product or service to an increasingly global market.

Hospices began with the mission of providing a superior service for a vulnerable population. The need for financial survival and growth came later. Early hospices were only concerned with finding a way to meet the needs of dying patients in a local community. As the hospice movement has grown and matured, the need to improve access to hospice care has driven concerns with financial viability, management efficiency, and acceptance by the mainstream medical community. Although it is good for hospices to improve their functioning, it should not be at the expense of their original purpose.

Some recent critics in the United Kingdom have questioned the continued relevance of the hospice movement. Colin Douglas (1992) has said, "The hospice movement is too good to be true and too small to be useful." He referred to the hospice movement as "deluxe dying for a minority" and expressed the most critical review by saying about hospice "Well done, thanks, and good-bye."

THE BUSINESS OF HOSPICE

Hospice care has become managed care. The reimbursement system for hospices in the United States at this writing is based on per diem payment. This is a set payment to the hospice for each day that a patient is enrolled in the program. Hospice is paid the set amount whether or not a direct service is provided that day. The hospice is responsible for making available a range of services and supplies for the terminally ill patient and family who enroll in the program.

These services include all necessary home care visitation services such as nursing, personal care, social work, therapies, counseling, and volunteer visits. Also included in the per diem payment is provision of all the medical supplies, treatments, durable medical equipment, diagnostic tests, labs, outpatient procedures, and any medications related to the terminal illness. These services need to be available or accessible to the patient and family 24 hours a day, 7 days a week, as determined by need.

Sometimes hospice is able to provide all these services to a patient and family for less cost than the amount of per diem received. If this happens, the hospice is able to keep the difference as a gain. For other patients and families, the cost of delivering all these goods and services is more than the amount paid. If this happens, the hospice loses money.

An analogy to this is that hospice is like an insurance company that must accept all applicants and cannot change the rate it charges. There is not a lot it can do to ensure that it is able to survive financially. Some of the decisions a hospice is forced to make to survive raise troubling questions. For instance, can a hospice decide not to admit a certain type of patient who is likely to require very expensive care?

Since the U.S. Hospice Medicare Benefit was established, hospices have operated in roughly the following way: The number of patients on whom hospice loses money should be less than those on whom it gains money. The belief was that if you cover the cost of some of the more expensive treatments, then physicians will refer more patients to you and you will benefit overall. The patients wanting fewer invasive interventions subsidize those who are more expensive to take care of.

As the health care system has attempted to reduce expenses and coverage, there seem to be more patients who are looking to hospice to cover more and more treatments, medications, tests, and so forth. This has in some cases upset this delicate balance and caused hospices to become more selective in patient admission. The point where access is difficult to determine continues to be the palliative–curative interface.

New developments in medicine and pharmacology are providing prolongative treatments to patients with fatal illnesses. These new drugs are not intended to cure the underlying illness or to relieve symptoms. They are specifically intended to delay death, usually by only weeks or months.

Examples of these new treatments include Riluzole for Lou Gehrig's disease, protease inhibitors for AIDS patients, and new oncologic treatments such as Taxol. These new drugs are very expensive and bring with them some ethical considerations. Is it life that is being prolonged or is it dying? Is this expensive use of limited health care resources just, when others are forced to receive little or no medical care?

These decisions need to be made in light of the individual patient's and family's values and goals. Too often treatments are continued or instituted simply because they are available. The assumption is that life must be continued because there is a means to do so. Hospice workers need to ask themselves whether the treatment has value for the patient.

Often it is the family who demands that treatment be continued. Too often this is insisted on for reasons that have nothing to do with what the patient wants. Family members do not want to feel guilty for not giving the patient a treatment that could offer some continued life or benefit. The exclusive focus on the primacy of the patient as health care decision maker ought to be rethought. Patients do not make health care decisions in a vacuum. They often make treatment decisions based on the feelings of family members.

So how is a hospice to make the right decisions about serving the needs of as many dying patients as possible without going bankrupt? A number of solutions to this problem have been tried as the hospice movement has matured.

These solutions include but are not limited to restricting access to some types of patients, serving patients under the home health agency model, and increasing size to help spread risk.

Some programs have attempted to limit the populations served by hospice to contain risk. For example, there are programs that will not admit a patient who is receiving any chemotherapy or radiation, even if it is specifically for symptom relief. This is usually done by the hospice with the position that patients must not be receiving curative treatment while in hospice. The NHO has taken the position that no one should be denied hospice care with such blanket exclusions (*Hospice Services: Guidelines and Definitions;* NHO, 1995b). It is the job of the hospice program to distinguish those palliative treatments from curative treatments.

Another patient population that hospices have had difficulty serving are people living with AIDS. So many of the new drug treatments are enormously expensive and so many young patients refuse to believe that they will die of the disease. This has led some programs to avoid efforts to reach out to people living with AIDS and to set unique and possibly discriminatory admission policies.

With the advent of Medicare-focused medical review, some programs have decided to stop admitting or to severely limit admission of all patients with non-cancerous terminal illnesses. A more rigorous evaluation of prognosis for the non-cancer patient is necessary, but if policies are intended to limit access to prevent the hospice from any exposure, then they are unjust. The great majority of hospices are interested in serving the needs of all dying patients, but some may be setting policy with only self-preservation or profit in mind.

A new approach to the problem is to create new models of service delivery or to adapt old ones. Before the Medicare Hospice Benefit was created, some hospices used existing sources of reimbursement for elements of hospice care such as home health agency payment for skilled nursing, home health aide, therapy, and social work visits. These payments covered a portion of hospice service costs but had significant restrictions. The patient had to be homebound, only the skilled services of a nurse or other professional were covered, no medications were paid for, psychosocial services were very limited, and inpatient care was excluded.

So far hospices have not had much success getting insurers to pay for services outside those covered under the Hospice Medicare Benefit. The future of hospice reimbursement may lie in hospice's ability to become more flexible in what it gets reimbursed for.

The majority of hospice programs in the United States serve a small number of patients each year. The average daily census is fewer than 50 patients. This is a small volume for the amount of overhead each hospice must carry. As the costs of delivering hospice care increase, programs must find ways to reduce expenses or to raise more financial support.

The trend is for programs to grow in size either through increased penetration of the population of terminally ill people or through acquisition or merger with other hospice programs. Increased size allows for better economies of scale, reduced costs through bulk purchasing, more ability to spread risks, and less overall overhead.

Along with increased size come new problems for the hospice. There may be less flexibility in meeting patient care needs, it becomes more difficult for the organization to function as a supportive community, and community support may diminish. Records and procedures become standardized, and processes become resistant to change. Employees feel they are part of a large company and do not know those with whom they do not work. The community perceives the hospice as a large successful organization with reimbursement funding and no longer sees it as a charitable institution that needs financial support.

These challenges can be effectively dealt with if the organization empowers its employees to continually improve the organization, supports self-directed work teams, and seeks to meet the unique needs of the community it serves.

MANAGED CARE

Because hospices under the Medicare/Medicaid benefit function as a kind of managed care provider, one would assume that hospice care would fit well into the emerging managed care systems. This is both true and false. It is true that hospices have learned to develop systems for managing and sharing financial risk. Hospices are ahead of the home health industry, which is still set up on a fee-for-service basis. Insurers ought to embrace hospices that are striving to help patients make good decisions about end-of-life care. Inappropriate care at life's end is one of the major factors in escalating health care costs. Studies such as the Lewin VHI Medicare cost analysis (NHO, 1995a) for hospice benefit patients have shown that hospice saves $1.56 for every Medicare dollar spent on hospice.

So why is managed care seen as a threat to hospices? There are a number of reasons that have been put forward. First, insurers want the least expensive alternative for the patient. Many times, case managers view home health as less expensive. If they pay per visit and limit the visits, they are likely to pay out less for professional services than giving the hospice a per diem that is paid each day whether a visit is made or not. They often do not take into consideration that the package of services covered in the per diem, unbundled, may well cost the insurer more than the hospice's fee.

At around $90 a day for hospice care at home, insurers may feel that they are paying too much. Home health visits may run around the same price per visit but are not paid daily; however, they do not include costs for equipment, medical supplies, medication, counseling, phone advice, and 24-hour-a-day availability.

The difficult fact is that insurers do not want to pay for these costs. They are ratcheting down the payments for home health as well as hospice. They perceive that there is overuse in the field, and they do not want to pay for things that families may provide out of their pockets or with their own sweat.

This brings me to the second main issue in managed care. Managed care prefers to control all aspects of the delivery of health care. They would rather have home health and hospice as part of their integrated health systems. This integrated health system is controlled through a capitated payment methodology. In a capitated system, there are just so many dollars allocated for care in the home, including hospice. The managed care provider will keep this utilization under control by delivering the care directly or by using providers who agree to deliver the care for a set amount.

In capitated systems, there is a set income of money per member per month. After profits and so forth, there is only so much allocated for specific types of care. A provider is guaranteed to receive that allocation no matter how much actual service is provided. If the care costs less to deliver than the allocation, the provider gets to keep the difference. If more care is needed than funds allocated, the provider has a problem.

This type of system works reasonably well for care that is delivered in large volumes and is not greatly expensive (e.g., doctors' office visits). People go to see their doctor fairly often and it does not cost a lot per unit of service. There is an incentive to get the patient's problem solved without running a lot of expensive diagnostics and follow-up visits. In this arrangement, the doctor's office becomes a cost center rather than a revenue center. The more visits and services, the less money the doctor makes.

Hospice care does not do as well in this type of system. In a large population, terminal illness is a relatively infrequent event. It can also be a very expensive event. The cost risks can be quite high. Even one very expensive patient can skew the arrangement to cause financial difficulty for the provider. Infrequent services such as hospice should not be capitated. A recent report out of Texas showed how capitation can have a negative impact on hospice. The capitated amount set out for hospice care resulted in the following. If the patient was under hospice care more than 12 days, the hospice program lost money. This creates an incentive that encourages last-minute referral and also creates barriers to hospice admission. Nonetheless, managed care seeks to capitate every cost in the health care system.

Large, seamless integrated health systems do not accommodate the local community hospice very well. There can be difficulty with the way they interface. There have been instances where patients who were good candidates for continued curative treatment have been referred for hospice admission. This may help the managed care provider's costs but is not in the patient's best interests. Nor is referring the patient who will die within hours or days.

Many of the emerging integrated health care systems are adding hospice care to their continuum of care. This is being done either through acquisition of existing programs or through new start-up of programs in urban areas. New programs are more difficult to add owing to the time involved in establishing a referral base and in building a well-functioning interdisciplinary team. Community- or home-health-agency–based programs are becoming more interested in securing their survival by becoming part of a larger entity.

The problem with integrated health care is that it is not yet really integrated. There is no sense of how each type of patient is best managed throughout a health care delivery system. What is really being managed is the cost of health care, not health care itself.

LEADERSHIP STYLE

Hospices tend to attract employees and volunteers who are very altruistic and demand a great deal of their leaders. The not-uncommon dictatorial style of management found in the business world is not easily tolerated in a hospice program. The values of a hospice ought to be found in its leaders. If a hospice values teamwork, integrity, service, and caring, then it would be hypocritical for the leaders to act unilaterally, with self-interest and financial gain in mind.

Leadership in a hospice program calls on individuals to act with utmost integrity. Hospice puts itself on a pedestal, per se, in that it claims implicitly to put service above self. Its leaders must do the same or those they lead will refuse to follow.

On the continuum of leadership from laissez faire to dictatorial, hospice leaders tend to be toward the middle. They try to function democratically but are better off making disputed decisions decisively than being unable to act.

James Autry (1991), in his book *Love and Profit: The Art of Caring Leadership*, spoke to the type of management style that may work best in a hospice. Autry showed that the external rules and regulations of management are useless unless the leader really cares about the work and the people who do it. He pointed out that all real power is given to those who manage by those who are being managed.

The authoritarian "wait until someone messes up and then pounce on them" style of management does nothing to further any enterprise. To improve morale, productivity, and success, you must really care about the people you work with, not manipulate them. Autry believed that the workplace can provide opportunities for spiritual and personal as well as financial growth.

Autry (1991) gave five guidelines for managers:

1   Avoid in-box management—stay in touch with employees regularly.
2   Care about yourself—you cannot motivate others unless your own battery is charged.
3   Be honest—if you care, you have to be willing to make critical appraisals as well as give compliments and set standards that are applied equitably.
4   Trust your employees—most management manages to make people feel mistrusted.

5   If you do not care about people, get out of management before it's too late; save your health and other people a lot of misery because the business of management is all about working with people. The policies and procedures are not important if you do not have your heart in it.

Max DePree carried forward a similar philosophy in his books *Leadership Is an Art* (1989) and *Leadership Jazz* (1992). He called leadership "liberating people to do what is required of them in the most effective and humane way" (p. 1). He saw the work relationship as a covenant between the organization and the people who work there. Effective leaders inspire people to see new possibilities.

Good leaders and managers are continually moving forward, not maintaining the status quo. If you are not continually reinventing your organization, then entropy is likely setting in. It helps to have a passion for management, to be truly excited about the possibilities of taking ideas and translating them into reality. It ought to give the same sense of satisfaction that an artist gets when creating an object of art.

It is easy to become weighted down by the uncertainties of the future, the overwhelming challenges that must be faced, and the sometimes petty concerns and conflicts of coworkers. Being effective as a hospice manager requires one to believe in the philosophy of hospice care, to believe in the people who are drawn to work in hospice, to trust people and be willing to delegate, and to maintain a sense of excitement about the possibilities that lie ahead. Managers must always be looking ahead to what is possible, not bogged down in the day-to-day details.

To make change happen, the locus of responsibility for problem solving must shift to the people working there. Solutions to the challenges facing any company do not reside in the executive suite. They are in the collective intelligence of employees at all levels who must use each other as resources. Rather than relying on a heirarchical organizational structure in hospice, it is more effctive to use a client-centered approach. Figure 7.1 diagrams the circular structure of a client centered approach. In this structure, the patient and family are the primary focus of everyones' efforts. The clinical staff have primary responsibility to care for them. In the next circle the administrative and operations staff forcus on making sure the clinical staff have the resources and support to meet the needs of the patient and family.

HOSPICE AS A COMMUNITY

Organizations use many metaphors to describe their functioning. The most popular seem to be based on sports. The team is most common and denotes a closely functioning unit under tight direction by a leader, the coach. It is competitive, always opposed to other teams, and strives to be victorious. Hospice workers describe themselves as team members, although the analogy is a poor one.

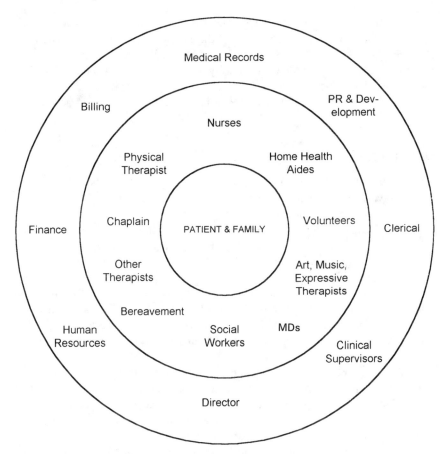

Figure 7.1   Client-Centered Organizational Chart

Hospice team members have no one to compete with. Their success does depend a great deal on cooperation and striving toward a common goal, but the goal is not to defeat anyone except, say, the effects of a terminal illness.

Another metaphor used is that hospice people are like family. They are close to each other and support each other through difficult times. Again, this analogy has difficulties. Everyone who works in a hospice comes from a different family. Each of those families has different dynamics. Some families can be very conflictual. Bringing family-of-origin issues to work can create all sorts of difficulties and can interfere with the ability to do what one is there to do.

A more helpful metaphor for hospice as a work group is a community. In a functioning community, each member has a distinct role that is needed for the community to operate successfully. Each role complements others and creates a kind of interdependence. There can be overlap as people cover for each other if needed in performing tasks.

In hospice, the total care of the patient is dependent on the efforts of each caregiver. If anyone fails to do their part there is an effect on all. For example, the care can be excellent for months, but if the on-call nurse fails to be there for the family when the patient dies, the family may remember only their disappointment at the last. The popular expression "It takes a village to raise a child" could also be modified to "It takes a community to care for a dying person."

VOLUNTEER ISSUES

Hospice care in the United States began through the efforts of volunteers. Many professional and lay people gave of their time and talents to create a new way of caring for dying people. The fact that people give of themselves to care for others has powerful significance to those who receive the care. People experience care given by those paid to provide care differently than they experience the same care given by a volunteer.

This observation has great significance for the success of the hospice movement. The extra dimension of caring provided by volunteers has always been one of the unique features of hospice care. It is also one of the features that has become hard to sustain. As funding for hospice care has increased, so have the paid staff needed to deliver the increased benefits of hospice care to an increasing number of people.

When hospices cared for a small number of patients at a time, volunteers could handle the load. Now there are hospice programs caring for thousands of patients at home on a given day. As volunteers nowadays are primarily people who also work, it is impossible for volunteers to be able to respond to all the needs of patients who depend on hospice for their care.

Another important dynamic here is that volunteers are less inclined to give when they know others are being paid to provide the same services. People in this society are very focused on remuneration and can be resentful if they feel they are being taken advantage of. Some volunteers give their time with the expectation that they will eventually be paid for their services when a position becomes available.

These issues have led to a situation where few volunteers are used in hospice in a professional capacity. The main role of the hospice volunteer in the United States is to be a support person who provides emotional support and practical assistance for the patient and family: to be a listener when a day has been hard, to be there to give respite so the family can get away to do errands, to drive to an appointment, or to help with the kids.

To the credit of the hospice movement, volunteers still play a very important role in caregiving, unlike other social movements begun by volunteers. A volunteer can be the most significant person to the dying patient. Volunteers often have more one-on-one time to spend with the patient and can become very close. They provide much of the hospitality of hospice.

STANDARDS AND ACCREDITATION

Standards

At the beginning of the hospice movement, there were few standards for how a hospice program ought to function, beyond those characteristics listed in chapter 1. Various standards have been put forward for hospice services. At the present time, the most comprehensive standards available in the United States for hospice care are the NHO's (1993) *Standards of a Hospice Program of Care.*

NHO's standards are divided into 11 chapters, including

- access to care
- patient/family as the unit of care
- hospice interdisciplinary team
- interdisciplinary team plan of care
- scope of hospice services
- coordination and continuity of care
- utilization review
- hospice services record
- governing body
- management and administration
- quality assessment and improvement

These standards were developed by the NHO Standards and Accreditation Committee to reflect the breadth and scope of state-of-the-art hospice care in the United States. The Standards and Accreditation Committee is made up of experienced hospice professionals from around the United States. Representatives of the hospice disciplines are included (nursing, social work, chaplaincy, education, medicine, management, and administration) and support is provided by NHO staff.

The standards are presented in a principal–standard–outcome format. Each chapter is introduced by a principle that reflects a fundamental tenet of hospice care related to that standard. Each standard is a norm that represents excellence in hospice practice. Outcomes are measurable results that are expected when a standard is applied and met. When not met, the outcomes give guidance as to what needs to be changed. NHO (1994a) has also published a companion *Standards of a Hospice Program of Care: Self Assessment Tool* that adds examples of compliance, showing how to comply with the standards in real-life terms.

The Access to Care chapter includes standards for how a hospice conducts community needs assessment, develops admission and discharge criteria, provides planned community education activities, does media promotion, and promotes cultural diversity. The Patient/Family as the Unit of Care chapter includes how hospices can promote family participation in provision of services, respect for patient–family values and beliefs, informed consent, advanced directives, explanation of rights and responsibilities, and support for primary caregivers.

The Hospice Interdisciplinary Team chapter includes standards that identify the members of the team and their qualifications. Included in this chapter is a standard that each member of the hospice team recognizes and accepts a fiduciary relationship with the patient and family. This means that hospice workers do not misuse their relationship of trust with the patient and family.

The Interdisciplinary Team Plan of Care chapter addresses the requirements for planning that go into the delivery of hospice care. The plan is interdisciplinary and individualized to the needs of the patient. A plan for bereavement interventions is also developed.

The largest chapter is Scope of Hospice Services, which includes a detailed description of what is required of the medical director, nurses, social workers, counselors, chaplains, and volunteers. There is also a detailed description of requirements for pharmaceutical services, pathology and laboratory, radiology, emergency medical services, access to medications, equipment, and supplies. The hospice must also address safety, emergency preparedness, and infection control and have a comprehensive bereavement service. Standards for home care delivery and facility based care are included.

The Coordination and Continuity of Care chapter explains what must be available 24 hours a day and how transfers must occur when the patient moves from home to inpatient care, or vice versa. How the hospice handles the transition if the patient is discharged is described. In the Utilization Review chapter, hospices are required to look at both the over- and underutilization of services as well as the appropriateness of admission and discharge.

The Hospice Services Record chapter details all the record-keeping requirements of the hospice. The Governing Body chapter gives all the requirements of governance, including planning, approval of policy, appointment of administrator, financial responsibility, evaluation of all activities, and avoidance of conflict of interest.

Under the Management and Administration chapter, standards define how roles, responsibilities, and accountability are assigned throughout the organization; how human resources are managed; how financial policies and practices are implemented; and how ethical dilemmas are handled. The final chapter, Quality Assessment and Improvement, asks hospices to assess and improve the quality and efficiency of governance, management, clinical, and support processes.

One of the current problems in the U.S. hospice community is the lack of consistency among hospices as to compliance with standards. The NHO standards are professional association standards. A member of NHO is expected to meet the standards, but there is no means of enforcement. Few hospices conduct self-assessment, let alone report their results.

Accreditation

In 1984, the JCAHO established an accreditation program for hospices. The accreditation standards were developed with extensive input from the hospice community. In 1990, JCAHO discontinued the program. Of the approximately 550 hospices accredited by JCAHO, only about 50 community- or home-health-agency–based hospices made the voluntary decision to become accredited. The remainder were hospital-based programs that had to be accredited because of their hospital ownership.

The bulk of the hospice community did not support the program with their participation. Many programs said that they already had to meet Medicare guidelines and questioned the value of accreditation. As a result, JCAHO was losing money and had pressure from the hospitals to discontinue the program.

In 1995, JCAHO decided to again offer accreditation to hospices. This time it would be as a part of the home health accreditation program. Many hospices pushed for a separate program. It was felt that making hospice a part of the home health program would reinforce the erroneous conclusion that home health and hospice were synonymous. Nonetheless, JCAHO went ahead with the program. Hospitals and home health agencies with hospice programs are generally required to be surveyed. This time it appears that more freestanding hospices are opting for accreditation. As networks of care are being formed, it is apparent that those without accreditation may be left out of the integrated care delivery systems that are being developed.

EXAMPLES OF PROBLEMS IN MANAGEMENT

What follows are some examples of real problems seen in starting and running hospice programs. It is hoped that the reader will use them as instructive examples to be avoided in the course of operating any organization.

A hospice program was started by a group of people, including a physician, who all volunteered their time. Funding was sought, and a nonprofit board of directors was formed. The physician became the medical director as well as chairman of the board. A group of community people were invited to be members of the board, including another local physician. In the course of developing programs and hiring staff, the director, who was inexperienced in management, was asked to hire as a nurse manager the former wife of one of the board members.

Time passed and the program grew. The nurse manager was ineffective in coordinating the clinical program, and the other staff began to complain to the director. The director tried to help the nurse manager to improve but was rebuffed. He began contemplating dismissal of the nurse manager and went to the medical director to discuss it. The medical director was against the idea.

The director went to a psychotherapist who had been hired to provide support to the patients as well as the staff and learned that the clinical manager and the medical director were having an affair. The director confronted the medical director about this but got no response. The director, realizing his predicament, decided it was probably best to leave the organization. Soon after this, at the chairman's suggestion, the board privately suggested that the director resign.

This example shows how dangerous it can be to confuse roles between the board and staff and to avoid dual relationships. Boards must avoid unethical self-serving actions. It is also a reminder that emotional entanglements can become a minefield in any organization.

The next example involves leadership style. A new hospice director was hired to run a community-based hospice that was a small, volunteer-based program. This director had a background in business and began working to establish the program on a sound financial footing. She gained Medicare certification for the program and greatly expanded the service area.

As funds came in, the program grew and more staff were hired. Each year, the fund balance grew and the organization saw a significant net profit. To maintain this level of financial performance, the director required the staff to justify all expenses. If a patient was hospitalized, the nurse case manager would be grilled about why this was needed (sometimes in front of coworkers). Any unusual expenses were questioned, and sometimes physicians were told they could not order tests or certain medications.

A rift grew between the office staff and the clinical staff. The office staff felt they were most important because they kept things organized and financed. The clinical staff felt they were most important because without them there would be no hospice care. They resented the emphasis on finances and intrusions into their clinical judgment. They wanted some appreciation rather than just criticism for things that they could not control.

The director felt she had enemies on the staff and sought to get rid of some individual staff. Finally, the situation came to a head, and most of the clinical staff resigned. The director decided the situation was too stressful and also resigned. The organization was left without leadership and with a demoralized staff.

Hospices are often started by charismatic leaders without the skill to build an organization. At this point, boards often bring in someone with a business background who succeeds in creating the necessary structure but who lacks the vision or values to carry the organization forward. It is relatively easy to set up a business structure. What is needed are leaders who can inspire the staff to grow and move forward with the organization.

We turn now from specific hospice management issues to some of the more general problems hospices face in our health care system. The Hospice Medicare Benefit has shaped much of the movement in the United States. We will explore the impact of the Benefit on hospice, as well as associated problems.

Chapter Eight

The Bureaucracy of Dying

"What tormented Ivan Illich most was the deception, the lie, which for some reason they all accepted, that he was not dying but was simply ill, and that he only need keep quiet and undergo a treatment and then something good would result."

—*The Death of Ivan Illich*, Leo Tolstoy

DEATH IN OUR HEALTH CARE SYSTEM

In the 1800s and 1900s in Sweden, just-married couples would visit the church graveyard to pick out a spot to bury their children who would not survive. High infant and childhood mortality was a fact of life, and few lived to a ripe old age. Thanks to advances in modern medicine, people can now look forward to an average life expectancy in the 70s. Although they may live longer, however, they may not enjoy the support of extended family that their ancestors did.

Today the family is barely able to take care of itself, let alone elderly infirm relatives. Most families, if intact, lack the ability to provide full- or part-time elder care. It is the norm for both husband and wife to work outside the home. The sense of bonding and acceptance of responsibility for parents seen in earlier generations is noticeably lacking in today's society. The proliferation of skilled nursing facilities for care of elderly and infirm persons is a testament to the breakdown in family and social structure.

In a recent Gallup Poll (NHO, 1992), Americans were asked where they would want to be cared for if they faced a terminal illness. Nine out of 10 people said they preferred to be cared for and to die in their own homes, and 3 out of 4 were very interested in hospice care when it was described to them. However, 22% of those who were interested in the services hospice programs provide said, when presented with the word *hospice*, that they were unlikely to choose it because they were unfamiliar with it.

THE MEDICARE BENEFIT

In the 1970s, American hospices were mainly organizations that survived on grants, donations, and volunteers. Professional nursing services were often provided by a local home health agency, if at all. Some hospices provided free nursing services or got licensed as home health agencies to receive reimbursement for home health. Emotional, spiritual, and practical support continued to be provided by volunteers.

Volunteer services by professionals were hard to sustain. As money was raised, there was pressure to pay for professional services. When one professional got paid, others were reluctant to donate their services. When professionals from other organizations were involved, it was difficult for hospice to be in control of the care delivered. Gradually, U.S. hospices had to find a way to finance their multidisciplinary operation.

In the United Kingdom, hospice care was provided by professionals from the start; there was less emphasis on lay volunteering. Funding came primarily from philanthropic sources. Nearly all care was delivered in an inpatient setting. Supporters could see bricks, mortar, and how care was being delivered. In 1995, only 38% of hospice expenses were paid for by the U.K. National Health Service.

In the United States, care was being delivered in the patient's home. Initial foundation and grant support was decreasing as hospices were no longer the new thing. Hospice leaders saw that for hospice care to grow and for comprehensive services to be delivered, there had to be an ongoing source of financial support. Because the health care system was funded through insurance reimbursement and most hospice patients were elderly and covered under the Medicare program, it made the most sense to develop a hospice Medicare benefit.

A national task force was formed to develop a model benefit proposal. The Health Care Finance Administration (HCFA) conducted a demonstration project to study the feasibility of reimbursing hospice care. In 1982, Congress created a Medicare benefit for hospice care. The NHO became a forum for debate on the pros and cons of government support for hospice care. Some believed that becoming part of the reimbursed system of health care would ruin the U.S. hospice movement. Others saw it as the movement's means for success.

Those who worried about creation of a hospice benefit feared that it would introduce bureaucracy into the movement. Limiting admission to 6 months seemed an arbitrary restriction. They realized that hospices would have to become professional organizations with all the accompanying structures and documentation. There was a fear that volunteers who were the mainstay of the movement would be shoved aside by professionals. Some felt that hospice care should not be paid for, that to introduce payment would contaminate the purity of providing selfless service to dying patients.

Others believed that hospice care would never become part of the health care system or be able to serve significant numbers of dying people without a reimbursement system. They argued that current hospice services lacked the professionalism and resources needed to deliver comprehensive services.

MEDICARE CERTIFICATION

Medicare Hospice Benefit regulations required a hospice to become certified before receiving reimbursement. Usually a state surveyor would visit the hospice to determine if all the "conditions of participation" in the program were met. These conditions included arrangements for a physician medical director, an administrator, and patient care coordinator. The hospice had to employ all "core" members of the hospice team, including nurses, social workers, medical director, and counselors. Bereavement follow-up with the families served had to be provided for at least 1 year. Hospice could either directly provide or contract for home health aides–homemakers; physical, speech, and occupational therapists; and inpatient care for symptom management and respite. In addition, the program had to provide for medical supplies, durable medical equipment, and medications. All these services had to be delivered if they were reasonable and necessary for the palliation and management of the terminal illness. Medical and nursing services, and other team services as needed, had to be available 24 hours a day, 7 days a week.

Hospices had to keep records, perform assessments, and develop and update plans of care. These updates were to occur at least every other week. Hospices had to provide education and in-service training for staff and volunteers. Volunteer activities had to comprise at least 5% of all services, and cost effectiveness had to be documented. The program had to conduct quality assurance activities and comply with all laws and regulations.

Levels of Care

Four levels of care are covered under the Medicare Hospice Benefit. Routine home care is the benefit if the patient is at home or in a nursing facility and receiving routine services. Continuous home care can be provided during periods of crisis. Anywhere from 8 to 24 hours of mostly skilled care can usually be paid for if it would keep the patient out of the hospital. The third level of care is inpatient respite. This is up to 5 days of inpatient care in a Medicare-certified acute or skilled nursing facility for the purpose of giving the patient's caregivers a rest. The fourth level of care is general inpatient care, which again is provided in Medicare facilities and is for active management of distressing symptoms of terminal illness.

The patient is entitled to two hospice benefit periods of 90 days, and an unlimited number of 60 day benefit periods. At the end of each period, the patient must be recertified as terminally ill. The patient is required to sign an election statement signifying that she or he chooses hospice care for management of the terminal illness in place of regular Medicare benefits. The hospice must also obtain the signatures of the patient's attending physician and the hospice medical director certifying that the patient has six months or less to live if the illness runs its normal course.

The Medicare Hospice Benefit was the only new service to be added to Medicare during the Reagan administration. It enjoyed widespread bipartisan support. At first, hospices did not embrace the program. Many believed it would create too many restrictions and requirements. Gradually, more and more hospices became certified for reimbursement. Those who were certified demonstrated that reimbursement allowed growth and an array of services that could not be provided by noncertified programs.

Growth

The growth of the patient population served by hospices in the past 10 years has been impressive. In 1985, when NHO did the first hospice census, 158,000 patients were served. The latest census conducted in 1996 revealed that 450,000 were served. Figure 8.1 illustrates the growth in hospice patient admissions. Average growth in patients served has been 13% in the 1990s.

In the 20-some years since the first hospice program began in the United States, there has been a rapid proliferation of program development. In 1996, NHO identified over 2,900 operating or planned hospice programs in all 50 states and Puerto Rico. Average annual growth of new hospices has averaged around 8% in the 1990s and has increased to about 13% in the past 5 years.

In 1994, 14.8% of all people who died in the United States from all causes were under the care of hospice programs. One in every seven Americans who died was served by a hospice. By 1996 that number had increased to one in five. In 1994, 36% of those who died of cancer received hospice care. Hospices have been trying to improve access for people with AIDS, and in 1994, 31% of people with AIDS who died in the United States also received hospice care.

Focused Medical Review

Until 1993, hospices received little scrutiny from HCFA. There was a perception that hospices were special providers who did not need to undergo the frequent audits other providers were put through. A couple of hospice programs in Puerto Rico were found to be signing up people for the hospice benefit who were not terminally ill. These incidents of apparent fraud caused HCFA to reconsider this

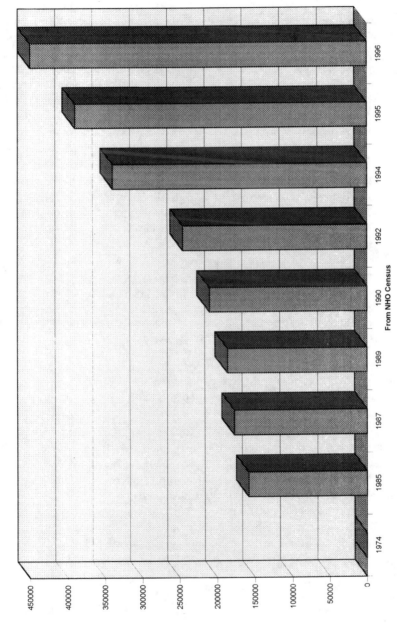

Figure 8.1 Growth in U.S. Hospice Patient Admissions

position and to suggest that intermediaries conduct audits to determine if hospices had unusually long lengths of stay.

Some of the Medicare intermediaries did look at hospice lengths of stay and discovered that a number of hospice patients remained on the benefit for unusually long periods. These were usually patients with non-cancerous terminal illnesses such as emphysema, congestive heart failure, or Alzheimer's disease. These are diseases that are especially difficult to prognosticate about. A heart patient may appear very close to death and in a few weeks be relatively stable. People with AIDS can go through a roller-coaster trajectory, coming near to death and bouncing back to baseline. In comparison, malignant diseases have a much more predictable course.

The Office of Inspector General and the Intermediaries have also grown concerned that there is some potential for abuse under the hospice benefit. Along with home health agencies and durable medical equipment suppliers, there is little oversight of what is actually being provided to Medicare recipients at home. The vast majority of hospice providers are reputable organizations that want to improve care of dying patients. However, there may be some who want to use hospice's good name to profit excessively.

Other areas of focus that are under government review include the following:

- engaging in marketing strategies that offer incomplete information about Medicare entitlement under the hospice benefit to induce patients to elect hospice
- encouraging hospice beneficiaries to temporarily revoke their election of hospice during a period when costly services, covered by the hospice plan of care, are needed for the hospice to avoid the obligation to pay for such services
- failure of hospices to notify prospective patients or their representatives that they will no longer be entitled to curative treatment if they elect hospice
- refusal by or failure of hospices to provide or arrange for needed care

There is also considerable concern about how the hospice benefit is provided to people in nursing homes. In some settings, there may be an inducement for the nursing home to refer patients to hospice and a duplication of services. If a hospice provides fewer services to a patient who is in a nursing home than they would provide to a patient at a personal residence, there could be a problem. In the future, there may be a reduction in reimbursement for hospice care in nursing homes to account for differences. Clearly, no one in the hospice movement wants providers who cut corners in patient care to increase profits.

THE PROBLEM WITH PROGNOSIS

Hospices were being asked to increase access to all dying patients at the same time as they were penalized if they made a wrong decision and admitted someone who did not die on schedule. Hospice relied on the judgment of physicians to predict prognosis. After all, what is a terminal prognosis other than a physician's judgment that someone has an incurable condition that will shortly result in death? What began to occur in 1994 was that Medicare insisted that hospices begin to be accountable for their decisions to admit patients. They could no longer rely just on a physician's judgment. Some physicians and patients and hospices had reason to want to access hospice's array of services not just for terminally ill patients but for chronically ill patients who were having trouble receiving services.

Hospices are specialists in comfort and management of distressing symptoms. Hospice staff were not used to playing the documentation games found in the rest of the health care system. Hospice nurses would document that the patient was having a good day, feeling all right. This was taken as evidence that the patient must not be dying. Sometimes the paradoxical could occur. A hospice might have a patient with chronic obstructive pulmonary disease who was near death at admission. Over the course of a few months, the hospice provides the patient and family with tremendous emotional and physical support and oxygen. The result of this good care is that the patient improves. The hospice discharges the patient, and he proceeds to go downhill and dies. In this not-too-uncommon scenario, hospice becomes a kind of life support for a patient who otherwise cannot get good care in the health care system. After a while, the hospice becomes fearful of discharging such patients.

When polled, physicians say they value hospice for the emotional support given to families. When a physician has been caring for a chronically ill patient for many years, she or he gets attached. The doctor also gets to feeling overwhelmed by the patient's emotional needs. It is easy to give over such patients to hospice whether or not they are really close to death. Patients view the hospice benefit as appealing. Current Medicare patients can become pauperized by all the copays and lack of coverage they experience during a chronic illness. The drug coverage benefit alone is motivation for many patients to enroll in hospice.

Some hospices came to rely on these chronically ill patients for financial survival. These are the patients for whom the hospice usually received much more reimbursement than needed. Actual cost of care for these patients was less than payment received. The hospice felt it needed these patients to cover the expense of admitting all those patients who were only in hospice a short time and cost more than the hospice was paid.

In this conflicted and confusing environment, there had to be a more honest and accurate way for hospices to decide which patients to admit and which might have to wait. When focused medical review of hospices began, HCFA realized that hospices were having a problem with accurate prognostication and that better tools were needed.

Prognostic Guidelines

The NHO (1995c, 1996b) offered to help develop guidelines that would assist HCFA, the intermediaries, and hospice providers to more accurately admit patients to the Medicare Benefit. As chair of the NHO Standards and Accreditation Committee, I was asked to put together a group to develop such guidelines.

In 1994, a group of physicians who had published or given presentations on prognosis in terminal illnesses were invited to join the task force. At first, the group assumed that the best method would be to develop a consensus based on expert clinical experience. Not much research on prognosis was being published in the hospice and palliative care literature.

The first draft of these guidelines was sent out for review to a selected group of hospice physicians. Expert physician opinion often varies. The task force realized that what was developed had to have a scientific basis to withstand government and professional review. The task force discovered that research on prognosis had become more popular recently and that some findings could be found in parts of the specialty medical literature. Many of the findings agreed with the experience-based guidelines that had been developed; others added new dimensions. To make the task manageable, the first version of the guidelines was limited to general factors affecting prognosis and disease-specific factors for endstage cardiac disease, endstage pulmonary disease, and endstage dementia. These three diagnoses covered the majority of patients admitted to hospices who were difficult to prognosticate about.

The *Medical Guidelines for Determining Prognosis in Selected Non-Cancer Diseases* (NHO, 1995c) was published by NHO and sent to Medicare payment intermediaries to use in claims and focused medical review. The second edition of the guidelines (NHO, 1996b) expanded the diseases covered (cardiac and pulmonary disease and dementia) to include HIV disease, liver disease, renal disease, stroke and coma, and amyotrophic lateral sclerosis.

No one knew if the guidelines would bring about a reduction in the number of patients served by hospices or an increase. The authors hoped that use of the guidelines would result in an increase in admission of appropriate patients to hospice.

Field testing of the guidelines is being planned, and NHO and HCFA have agreed that they will be modified as necessary as new research is reported. HCFA is exploring use of the guidelines as a tool for medical review of hospice appropriate claims. A new task force has been formed in 1997 to develop prognostic guidelines for cancer patients.

REIFICATION OF HOSPICE

In a recent lecture by the sociologist David Clark (1995), Max Weber's theory on the development of religion and the life course of a social movement was used to examine the genesis of the hospice movement. Weber used the religious metaphor to characterize how social movements progress from sect to denomination to church.

In the sect phase, the current world is rejected. Charismatic leaders produce key writings. For the hospice movement, people like Cicely Saunders, Elisabeth

Kübler-Ross, Herman Feifel, Robert Fulton, and John Hinton are examples of leaders who rejected society's taboo on discussion of death well before it became popular to do so. Classic books such as *On Death and Dying* (Kübler-Ross, 1969), *The Meaning of Death* (Feifel, 1959), *Death and Identity* (Fulton, 1965), and *Dying* (Hinton, 1972) gave hospice pioneers a kind of permission to push the boundaries of what was permissible.

Hospice in the United States entered the denominational phase in about 1983 with the creation of the Hospice Medicare Benefit. About this time, the movement started compromising with the world and began attempting to be respectable. The NHO began to grow, and JCAHO started developing its accreditation program. New services began to proliferate.

It is debatable whether hospice has reached the church stage. In the United Kingdom, hospice and palliative care do seem to be legitimate and have become part of the medical establishment. Some there are in favor of dropping the word *hospice* in favor of palliative care. In the United States, hospice is widely respected but not embraced by the leaders of the medical establishment. Work in palliative care is gaining some respect but is still not thought to be at the cutting edge of science.

Although hospice in the United States is still viewed as new, it does seem to be viewed by many in the euthanasia debate as one of the more conservative elements. Hospice does not seem to be willing to take as many of the risks it used to routinely face. A possible measure of the onset of entropy was suggested by David Clark (1995), who said that when "regurgitive conferences" begin to emerge, a new social phenomena may be stagnating.

All social institutions undergo a process of reification. That is to say, they gradually form boundaries and rules that define both what the institution is and what it is not. This is a process that gives the entity both definition and clarity while hardening it into something that is much more difficult to change. Where hospices were initially fluid and creative in their responses to the needs of dying patients in their communities, they are now concerned more with survival, consistency of care, and efficiencies of management.

ARROGANCE OF HOSPICE

Those who work in hospice care view their field as unique. No other health care provider is seen as quite as dedicated or caring or in tune with its patients' needs. Some in the field believe that hospice care is a model for the interdisciplinary delivery of care to all medical patients. Clinical experts in the field have often made overarching statements about hospice's ability to manage all symptoms of the dying process and that no patient has to ever die in pain. The problem, from hospices' perspective, is that not all patients are allowed to access hospice care. If they were, dying would always be a satisfactory and potentially rewarding experience.

Although hospice care has been shown to improve the quality of care for dying patients and their families, it is not for everyone. And although hospices have pioneered the best in palliative care procedures, there are some patients whose symptoms defy all interventions. Yes, patients can be sedated if their symptoms are too unbearable, but is this the same thing as a pain-free death? Hospices must recognize and come to grips with their limitations if they are to improve and take their place in the existing health care system. They must also accept the role of being a niche in the system and realize that hospice care may not be the model for all health care delivery systems.

The interdisciplinary care model is a breakthrough in the treatment of patients with complex medical problems. For an acute emergency room patient, however, the need is for decisive physician-directed intervention. For the patient with a single ailment, primary care will ordinarily suffice. The health care system cannot afford to attend to the medical, emotional, and spiritual needs of all patients.

At a time when the health care system is just becoming interested in end-of-life care, the hospice movement's response is that it is the answer. Just give all these patients hospice and there will not be a problem. This attitude does not help others to learn more about care for the dying. Also, *hospice,* as defined by the Medicare Hospice Benefit, is not for all people facing death. Hospices need to share what they have learned about caring for the dying with the rest of the health care system for major changes to occur in the care of all the dying. The hospice movement has failed to provide the leadership needed to fundamentally change the way people die in the United States. The hospice community seems to believe that end-of-life care belongs to hospice. There are many others who have a legitimate interest in the care of the dying and who need to be partners with hospice in developing a working system that meets the needs of those nearing the end of life.

The tendency toward arrogance is often reinforced by families who are in awe of the hospice workers' abilities to help them face death. Time after time, families tell the hospice staff and volunteers that they could not have survived the experience without hospice. After a while, staff and volunteers begin to believe that they really must be rather special.

It certainly is rewarding when the people one serves express appreciation; however, there is a danger here. Some in hospice work tend to have a need for such praise. When it is not forthcoming, there can be disappointment, and for those families incapable of appreciation, there can be disdain. After all, remember, it is not hospice workers' needs that are important here. Hospice can do its best work when there is honest humility in the care provided. It is more therapeutic for hospice to take a backseat to the family's role in caregiving.

Many families need very little from hospice other than empowering them to provide care and to communicate openly. Lao T'su (Blakney, 1955) spoke wisely when he said,

A leader is best when people barely know he exists,
not so good when people obey and acclaim him,
worst when they despise him.
Fail to honor people, they fail to honor you.
But of a good leader, who talks little
when his work is done, his aim fulfilled,
They will all say, we did this ourselves.

The bulk of the work of caring for dying patients is done by the family. Hospice provides them with the crucial training and support they need to accomplish this. It is really the family who deserve the credit and praise. It is more therapeutic to direct the attention to them as they will have less difficulty in bereavement if they believe their work made a difference in how their loved one died (Connor, 1996a).

Hospice patients face some of the most complicated medical management problems found in the health care system. However, as a managed care provider there is a disincentive to use outside consulting resources. It is not uncommon for hospice patients to have complex wound or stoma care requirements, yet there are very few hospices that have access to an enterostomal therapist. Hospice program philosophy stresses high-touch, low-tech care. Patients and families do better with less complex treatment options. However, there are some patients whose symptom management could be greatly enhanced through high-tech interventions.

The hospice community varies considerably in its medical sophistication. On one extreme are programs that refuse to do any "intrusive" interventions, such as IV fluids. On the other extreme are hospices that set no limits on the types of treatments administered, including total parenteral nutrition, resuscitation, or experimental chemotherapy.

The difficulties here are both philosophical and pragmatic. Hospice promotes the principle of autonomy. Patients have the right to choose whichever treatments they wish. However, when hospice disagrees with these choices, there is a problem. Hospice care is palliative care, yet how far can the notion of palliation be stretched? Many oncologists believe that nearly all the care they provide is palliative in that it will not cure the patient. Yet does it promote relief from distressing symptoms? Sometimes yes, sometimes no.

Arrogance comes into play when hospice thinks it knows what is best for the patient. People make choices for many complex reasons, both conscious and unconscious. The patient's goals are the patient's goals. The best hospice can do is help to understand and articulate them. Well-developed hospice programs try to do this around the time of entry into the program to avoid confusion. However, people are entitled to change their minds, and they often do.

Greatly limiting the choices patients can have in hospice leads to reduced access to hospice care. Removing all limitations to treatment in hospice leads to hospice care that is indistinguishable from care provided in the rest of the health care system. Hospice can bring its knowledge of how best to manage care at the end of life to patients, families, and physicians, but it has to accept their decisions and goals as right even if it disagrees.

QUALITY OF CARE

Is hospice care better than traditional care? Can quality of living or dying be measured? What are the measurable outcomes of hospice care? These and other questions have yet to be answered but must be addressed. Much of what has been described as unique to hospice care is difficult to measure.

The vast majority of hospices in the United States do not conduct research. Most programs are small and lack the expertise necessary to carry out investigations. More important, there is a general reluctance to involve patients in any activities that involve outside people. The privacy of patients and families is carefully guarded. Outside researchers are viewed as intruders who only add annoyance to people already stressed as a result of their circumstances.

On top of this, there is an unwillingness to consider using randomization when studying hospice care. It would be unethical for some patients to be denied access to hospice so that the effects of hospice could be studied. Because the randomized controlled design is the gold standard in science, it is very difficult for nonrandomized results to be accepted as definitive.

The health care system is moving toward agreed-on systems for measuring quality of care. The JCAHO has developed a system for providers to submit comparative performance data. The national HEDIS project is attempting to establish agreed-on outcomes for different health care providers. The NHO is just beginning to attempt standardization of data for consumer satisfaction and pain control (see chapter 12). At present, there is no agreed-on way of addressing other symptoms, let alone psychological or spiritual services.

PAUCITY OF RESEARCH

The hospice movement is now more than 30 years old. Many books have been written and there are a number of journals being published. What is striking is the lack of serious research being done in the field of palliative care in the US. Many of the studies that are published are small in scale or lack methodological sophistication. There has been very little funding in the United States for research in palliative care.

There was a demonstration project funded in the 1970s by the HCFA to examine the feasibility and cost effectiveness of hospice models (Greer, Mor, Morris, Sherwood, Kidder, & Birnbaum, 1986), and the National Institutes of Health recently funded development of pilot physician training programs in hospice and palliative care. There have been no Requests For Application to study improvement in the care of terminally ill persons despite the fact that cancer may soon surpass heart disease as the leading cause of death in the United States.

Since President Nixon declared a war on cancer in 1971, the United States has spent some $30 billion on cancer research. Scientists have made great progress in understanding how different types of cancer occur and are more sophisticated at tracking its course. However, treatment advances have had minimal impact on mortality rates. Physicians still cut cancer out with surgery, poison it with chemotherapy, and burn it with radiation.

There are a few attempts to stimulate research being developed. The Project on Death in America recently funded a variety of projects to look at end-of-life care and also funded a group of scholars. The National Hospice Foundation is attempting to raise funds to support research in hospice care. The Robert Wood Johnson Foundation is also interested in funding projects that improve understanding of end-of-life care and recently initiated the "Last Acts" program to change social attitudes toward care of the dying (see Organizational References).

All in all, research in care of the dying has not been viewed as important by the scientific community. The important work is in areas of high-tech care aimed at prolonging life. Oncogene research, AIDS treatment, and rescue chemotherapy are the new fields. Never mind that the overall cancer death rate has dropped slightly and while everyone waits for the elusive definitive cancer treatment, hundreds of thousands suffer both from treatment and disease.

PHYSICIAN INVOLVEMENT

The hospice movement was founded by physicians and other health care providers who were dissatisfied with the way dying patients were cared for. Today, the success of a particular hospice largely rests with how it is viewed by the medical community. Most physicians begin with a bias toward continued disease treatment.

The Hippocratic oath, emotional involvement with the patient, and medical economics all push against acknowledging that a disease is incurable. Recommending hospice care means having to openly acknowledge that the physician has been unable to cure the disease. This seems like a failure to many physicians who are sworn to work toward healing the patient. In addition, doctors become emotionally involved with many patients. When the patient becomes seriously ill, they focus more attention and concern on their welfare. Failure of medical therapeutics becomes a personal failure. It is human to feel they have let the patient down.

On top of all this are financial considerations. In the U.S. fee-for-service medical care system, the more medical care delivered, the more payment the physician receives. Many specialists, lacking the intensity of emotional involvement with the patient of the primary care physician, have a powerful financial incentive to continue treating the patient even when cure is unlikely. The movement toward managed health care changes this formula so that physicians are penalized if patients are overtreated.

How does hospice fit into all this? Some physicians view hospice as a great relief to the burden of supporting the patient emotionally; others see hospice as a symbol of their failure or as a competitor. These attitudes determine how local physicians will choose to use or not use a particular hospice program. It is possible for a hospice to change these perceptions, but it will require the right kind of education and experience. Education provided by other physicians is most effective, and positive experience working with the hospice is critical. If the physician hears from other respected colleagues that the program has helped and from patients and families that have been well served, some of the most ardent critics can be won over.

All of this occurs in the context of a health care system that does not value palliative care. Most physicians view the important work of medicine as efforts to cure or control the major diseases. Genetic research, transplantation, and pharmaceutical advancement are the areas of appeal for scientists and physicians.

The magic of overcoming mankind's perennial ills is appealing enough but added to this are enormous financial incentives. The newest treatments, equipment, and expertise are often the most rewarded. The health care system in the United States is fundamentally a business, and a hugely profitable one at that.

In contrast, the relief of suffering comes in a poor second, if that. Yet is this lack of interest and funding for palliative care appropriate given reality in the health care system? Each year in the United States, approximately 555,000 people die of malignant disease. Of these, a large percentage will experience severe pain. All will likely experience distress related to their disease or treatment. Add to this approximately 1,500,000 patients who die each year from other chronic diseases such as obstructive pulmonary disease, heart disease, dementias, motor neuron diseases, and the like.

Should vast sums continue to be provided to fund research into curative treatment and the investigation of treatment aimed at relief of suffering be neglected? At least some significant funding should be directed toward the science of palliative medicine.

In the United Kingdom, palliative medicine has been accepted by the Royal College of Medicine as a recognized subspecialty. Posts in palliative medicine have been created throughout the country to serve the needs of the terminally ill population. Curriculums have been developed for physician training, and research is encouraged. In the United States, the overabundance of specialists has discouraged the establishment of a subspecialty in palliative medicine. A lack of regard for the importance of symptom management and a lack of support from the Brahmins of the U.S. health care system make it questionable whether palliative medicine will ever become a specialty.

HEALTH CARE REFORM

In recent years, both major political parties in the United States have attempted to reform the health care system. In 1994, the Democratic Party tried to revamp the entire system, and in 1995 the Republican Party focused on the Medicare Program. Both efforts have focused on promotion of managed care and managed competition.

It is interesting to note that the Hospice Medicare Benefit was an experiment in managed care. The payment of a per diem for a package of health care services was a new way of shifting risk from Medicare to the provider. On the continuum of risk, there is less provider uncertainty than with capitated payment, but it is not a risk-free fee-for-service payment like the rest of the Medicare program.

Hospice then ought to be a good fit for managed care. Hospices are used to having to manage and share risk. Therefore, health care reform is seen as good for the hospice movement. However, it is not as simple as it seems.

As the managed care industry has developed in the United States, the primary emphasis has been on cost. Providers who can deliver care for the least expense are those who are given contracts and referrals. Quality has been a secondary consideration. These initial cost-driven decisions have resulted in some serious problems in health care delivery and satisfaction. The emphasis is shifting to value. Providers must be able to provide a service that is both effective and inexpensive. Consumers must be able to access the service and find it responsive to their needs.

Those providers who are willing to share the most risk with managed care partners are most attractive. This requires the ability to find ways of controlling expense without sacrificing quality. As the managed care system matures, it is focusing more on the outcomes of care. Providers who are able to demonstrate that they can achieve the best outcomes at the lowest cost are most likely to survive.

PROFIT VERSUS NONPROFIT HOSPICE

Modern hospice care began in the United Kingdom as a charitable enterprise. The Polish patient who left 500 pounds to Dame Saunders to start St. Christopher's Hospice near London did so as a charitable gesture. For the most part, hospice care in the United Kingdom continues to be funded by philanthropic support.

In the United States, early hospices were all begun as not-for-profit organizations. There was no funding other than donations and volunteer labor. The first hospice to change over to for-profit status was Hospice Inc. in Florida. They observed that for hospice to grow, capital was needed. They felt the best way to attract capital was to allow investment. It is important to note that the average hospice is still quite small (average daily census of fewer than 30 patients). Hospice Inc. changed its name to VITAS to emphasize a commitment to a broader range of care to patients at the end of life. This company is the largest provider of hospice care in the United States, with an average daily census in 1995 of 5,000 patients at 31 sites.

The great majority of hospices are still charitable organizations. Should hospices remain charities? This is a complex issue. The not-for-profit hospice has the following positive aspects. It does not have stockholders to satisfy and make a profit for. It is more reliant on and part of the community it serves. Charitable hospices tend to provide more services for their communities (i.e., support groups, counseling and bereavement follow-up, education programs, trauma services, camps). They tend to make more use of volunteers and to respond to local unique needs.

The downside of nonprofits are their relative lack of efficiency and organization. There is a tendency to stay with the familiar and to resist growth. There is little financial incentive to grow, and with increased size come challenges that many managers are not prepared to respond to. The result is often that difficult populations are not served.

For-profit hospices have found a foothold in metropolitan areas where significant populations have gone unserved. If the existing hospice does not respond quickly when hospital discharge planners need help with the disposition of an inpatient, they will give their business to someone who will.

Potential advantages of for-profit hospices include a tendency to be more efficient and able to change. They are more likely to be bigger as they do not owe their allegiance to a particular community. Having more capital available, they can develop or provide a wider range of programs (i.e., inpatient, nursing facilities, pharmacy, home health, residential care).

Drawbacks to for-profit hospice care can be conflict of value over the true mission of the organization; inability to develop viable volunteer services; a tendency to focus on core income-producing services instead of the actual needs of the population. A larger societal issue is whether it is appropriate for funds designated for health care to be siphoned off to pay shareholders.

Some say that there is really no difference between for-profit and not-for-profit organizations in that they both actually strive to produce a profit. The only difference is how the profit is used. Certainly some not-for-profit organization have done better at producing higher net incomes than for-profit corporations.

The for-profit versus not-for-profit difference may ultimately be less critical. The most important issue is the true purpose of the organization. If the purpose of the hospice is to effectively meet the needs and exceed the expectations of as many dying patients as possible, then it is doing its job. If it is not, then it should move aside.

CASE ILLUSTRATION

George

George was a 68-year-old patient with chronic obstructive pulmonary disease who was admitted to hospice in bad condition. He was continuously short of breath and could not ambulate or do personal care without assistance. He lived with a daughter who worked and could not stay with him. Our plan of care included assisting with personal care, nursing support, counseling, home equipment, and 24-hour support. After a few months, George seemed to be improved. He was breathing easier and had more energy. We continued to work with him, and he was quite open about preparing emotionally for death.

This situation continued for more than a year, and hospice personnel began to wonder if George was really terminally ill. We had his physician assess him, and we all concluded that he had improved but remained with an uncertain prognosis. After a few more months, we came to believe that George could continue like this indefinitely. We began to make arrangements to discharge him from the hospice program. We had ample time to say good-bye and made alternate arrangements to help with his personal care.

Everyone tried to make the best of the situation, but George was sad. It seemed as if he felt he had failed us in some way. The family was instructed to call us if his situation changed, and we stopped coming. Everyone wondered how George would do, and his nurse called a few times to check.

A few months passed, and one day we had a call from his daughter: George was much worse, could we come out? His nurse went right out and found George to be close to death. Hospice services were resumed, and staff helped care for him over the next 2 days. He died peacefully in his bed at home.

Afterward, everyone felt awful. We felt somehow we had contributed to his death by discontinuing services. In some ways, hospice became a kind of life support for George. The constant attention to his physical health and emotional well-being had kept him going. Without hospice, he felt he was a burden to his family. This is one of the paradoxes of hospice care; with good care many patients can actually live longer than they might otherwise have.

The business of hospice care is difficult enough. Added to this is society's disavowal of death. In the next chapter, the denial of death that is ingrained in today's culture is examined.

Chapter Nine

Society in Denial

"I'm not afraid to die. I just don't want to be there when it happens."

—Woody Allen

The effectiveness of hospice in helping patients and families face death is profoundly affected by their ability to face reality. Each patient and family comes to this ordeal with differing amounts of inner resources. Families vary enormously in their coping ability. Some can face adversity with tremendous strength, and others collapse or fall apart. Some refuse to believe the diagnosis will result in their death and fight to the bitter end; others fight for awhile but tire and give in to their deaths.

The dynamics of hope and denial are a universal part of the experience of facing death. All people want to hope for the best and believe that they will be the 1 out of 20 who makes it. It is a normal and healthy part of the reaction to news of a life-threatening illness to refuse to believe that it is really happening. A person thinks, there must have been a mistake, the reports got mixed up, it just can't be me, this only happens to other people!

After enough time has passed, it begins to sink in: This really is happening, I could die of this disease. This process does not happen the same way for everyone. Some persist in the belief that a mistake was made or minimize the seriousness of the situation. Why is it that so many people rail against the inevitable? Why do they have so much trouble accepting the reality that they can die?

ARE WE A DEATH-DENYING CULTURE?

Throughout history, man has attempted in many ways to defeat death. The ancient Egyptians saw death as a journey to a new land. The dead person was buried with provisions to aid in the long journey. The physical body was carefully preserved so it would stay intact. Valuable items were left in the tomb so that one's station in this life could be maintained in the next. All this was in the vain belief that death was not really death.

Most religions attempt to reassure people that there is a continuity to life and that death is not the end of one's individual existence. Modern medicine views death as the enemy to be defeated no matter what the cost. There is an implicit message that life can and should be prolonged no matter what the consequences. In the past 50 years, there has been so much progress in the treatment and cure of disease that society has come to see death as an unwanted unnatural consequence and someone's fault.

In this same time span, death has gone from being a part of the fabric of life at home to a far-removed event that happens in hospitals and institutions. Youth is worshiped, and old age and death are banished. People protect their children from death by making them stay home from funerals and use euphemisms for death such as *passing away, resting,* or *gone away.*

When someone does die, it has to be because someone made a mistake somewhere. It must be someone's fault, the doctor or the hospital or the ambulance or the insurance company. This society is the most litigious in the world. U.S. citizens file twice as many lawsuits per capita as do people in other industrialized countries. People refuse to accept that sometimes death just happens in spite of everyone's best efforts.

It is still universal practice in hospitals that all patients must be resuscitated in the absence of a DNR order. Of course, most people would want all efforts to be made to save them if they had a reversible condition. This is more the exception than the rule in acute hospitals, however. Those resuscitated are predominately chronically and terminally ill people who will not recover in spite of the resuscitation attempt. For all patients 60 years and older only 10–17% survive after arrest and for those with a chronic condition and poor prognosis, the survival rate is 0–5% (Murphy, Burrows, Santilli, Kemp, Tenner, Kreling, & Teno, 1994).

The United States is both a death-denying and death-obsessed culture. Its people are obsessed with unnatural death but avoid natural death. The media are saturated with unnatural death. Violence, mayhem, and destruction are the staples of television, movies, and fiction. People lose interest in anything that lacks violent or romantic content.

In contrast, it is rare to find entertainment that addresses natural dying. When a show does attempt to deal with the subject, it is usually considered too serious or depressing. Surprisingly, some of these efforts have left strong impressions (e.g., the movie "Brian's Song"). People recoil from reminders that they must experience their own personal deaths. It is easier to distance themselves from death when it is happening to someone else, especially someone they dislike.

The growth of the hospice movement is greatly affected by the tendency to want to avoid facing the reality of an incurable condition. Hospice has been set up in such a way that patients must renounce further attempts at curative treatment. They must acknowledge being informed of the diagnosis and prognosis and make the shift to palliative care. In spite of all the wonderful services and support that hospices have to offer, this is a difficult thing to face. By forcing people to face reality and their own denial, hospices may have significantly limited their ability to serve to serve those most in need of help.

THEORIES OF DENIAL

The idea of denial originated in the early writings of Sigmund Freud (1924). He introduced the term *disavowal,* meaning a refusal of reality. He originally thought of this as a symptom of psychosis but later came to view it as a mechanism of defense (Freud, 1940). Anna Freud (1948) saw denial as a necessary component of all defensive operations. Psychoanalytic thinkers view denial as the result of intrapsychic conflict. For a terminally ill person, the external threat of death can cause a person to feel in danger of being overwhelmed with anxiety. An individual who lacks higher functioning defenses resorts to the more primitive use of denial to survive emotionally (see Sjoback, 1973, for a more thorough account of the development of the psychoanalytic concept of denial).

Other writers have viewed denial as a more adaptive coping process (Beilin, 1981; Beisser, 1979; Dansak & Cordes, 1978–1979; Haan, 1965; Hackett & Cassem, 1970) or as a helpful strategy in the early stages of response to cancer (Detwiler, 1981; Falek & Britton, 1974; Kübler-Ross, 1969; Weisman, 1972).

Other researchers have seen both negative and positive functions for denial in seriously ill and elderly people. Becker (1973) attempted to explain the inability to deal with death through Otto Rank's depth psychology of heroism and its failure. A hero faces death without denial. This society has failed to incorporate the values of the hero.

Weisman (1972) proposed three degrees of denial. First-order denial is obvious denial of the main facts of the illness: "Who, me? I don't have cancer!" Second-order denial is denial of the significance or implications of the illness: "Sure, I have cancer, but it's no big deal." Third-order denial is refusal to believe the illness will result in death: "Yeah, I have cancer and it's serious, but I'm not going to die." Such people will believe that they can remain in their incapacitated state indefinitely.

Breznitz (1983) expanded on Weisman's (1972) three degrees by proposing seven different kinds of denial. They are each related to a different stage in the processing of threatening information. The seven include denial of

- information
- threatening information
- personal relevance
- urgency
- vulnerability
- effect
- affect relevance

In Breznitz's view the more denial used, the more reality distortion is present.

A significant association between denial and preservation of significant relationships was observed by an associate of Weisman's named Hackett. Hackett (Hackett & Weisman, 1964, 1969) observed how denial arose within the social sphere. Hackett proposed a scale (Hackett & Cassem, 1974) that classified deniers into three groups: mild, moderate, and major. Those in the major category would never acknowledge a fear of death, whereas those in the mild category were readily fearful and lacked consistent defenses against their anxiety. Most were classified in the moderate category. Hackett noted, however, that the criteria were never precise.

From the field of stress and coping, Richard Lazarus has contributed a great deal to the literature on the use of denial. Lazarus and Golden (1981) suggested that age is an important factor in response to terminal illness and that older people tend to use denial less. They suggested the term *denial like processes* to show that what may appear to be denial is not what one thinks it is. They concluded that "denial like processes can have both beneficial and harmful consequences depending on the timing, circumstances, and pervasiveness." Lazarus and Golden's concept of cognitive appraisal helps researchers understand that people will vary greatly in their reactions depending on how they evaluate the significance of the threat to their well-being. This can help researchers understand the variety of emotional responses seen in those facing death.

A more recent author (Taylor, 1989) explored the adaptive use of positive illusions. These are the sometimes self-deceptive ways people help get themselves through difficult crises. "Repression and denial alter reality whereas illusions simply interpret it in the best possible light."

DENIAL AND ACCEPTANCE

Denial and acceptance are usually thought of as two points on a continuum of how people respond to dying. Denial is the least adaptive response, and acceptance is the most adaptive. This is certainly an oversimplification of a very complex dynamic.

Elisabeth Kübler-Ross (1969) put forward one the first theories to explain how people respond to the knowledge of impending death. Her stage theory begins with denial, which functions as a psychic shock absorber that gradually gives way to anger at the reality of the situation. This is followed by bargaining with God to live and, when this does not work, depression at one's helplessness. Finally, the person reaches acceptance, which is characterized by a turning away from life and giving in to death. Kübler-Ross's observations were never intended to be cast in stone or to be taken as the only way people face death; however, people tend to want to simplify difficult subjects and have misinterpreted her work.

A number of authors have criticized the whole notion of stage theories of dying (see chapter 4). One's response to the knowledge of impending death is not linear. It is distinguished by vacillations in emotional and cognitive response. The most common response is ambivalence. The person simultaneously hopes for a cure while he or she wishes for release. People want either to beat the disease and return to their previous existence or to have it over with. It seems that being in the limbo of neither living nor dying is the least tolerable. Avery Weisman (1972) referred to this state as "middle knowledge," or the chronic living–dying interval. In spite of the popularity of Kübler-Ross's (1969) model, there really is no well-recognized succession of emotional responses that is typical of people facing death.

In spite of this, there are some people who seem to face death with clarity and openness. They seem to accept the fact that they are dying and see no need to struggle over it. This sometimes occurs after unpleasant initial reactions or may just as likely be their reaction from the beginning of their knowledge that death is near. It is difficult to know why some people face death with an inner peace and others fall into fear or avoidance.

When acceptance is seen in a dying person, it has variously been described as a kind of peace that came upon the person or a withdrawing from life and worldly things. It is a less-than-common response that caps an exceptional life. It is not the resignation often seen in someone who says "What else can I do?" or "I want to die and get it over with." Resignation is a kind of learned helplessness. The anger, attempts at control, and other responses have not changed the relentless course of the disease. It is no longer possible to maintain denial in the face of decline. At least enough time has passed to gather the strength to face reality.

One might see acceptance in the above. Being able to face the reality of one's death without being overwhelmed emotionally is a considerable accomplishment. But there is something different about the quality of acceptance. It is more than just giving up and turning away. It is perhaps a curiosity about what lies ahead, a sense of completion, a feeling that one's life has been accomplished and one's work has been done. It is to be in awe of the inevitable miracle about to happen. It is a profound understanding that life goes on without one and that everything will be all right; one is not essential to the continued functioning of the rest of life.

INTERPERSONAL AND INTRAPSYCHIC DENIAL

When one thinks of denial in the face of death, one thinks of a person who cannot face reality. One assumes that the person is so devastated that he or she must resort to a primitive defense that blocks out the obvious reality. The person's persistent denial is evidence of serious psychological disturbance, an almost psychotic refusal to face reality that will have serious consequences.

Although this may sometimes be the case, it is probably the exception rather than the rule. It has been suggested that what is usually thought of as denial is more often a conscious decision to present a more optimistic picture. This is done in the belief that it will preserve interpersonal relationships that are necessary for coping. People are afraid that if they speak truthfully about how they feel it will drive their loved ones away. Unfortunately, the opposite is usually the case; when people do not talk openly about their fears and feelings, those around them are uncomfortable and tend to become more distant.

The notion that most denial is based on interpersonal relations is consistent with experience in hospice and has been documented in the literature (Connor, 1994). Denial may be used for a number of relational reasons. People may wish to protect their loved ones from the distress they may imagine their loved ones will suffer if they must confront the reality of their dying. They may feel guilt over their condition and the distress it causes others. A dying person may fear abandonment by those closest to him or her if dying is discussed openly.

In contrast to denial for interpersonal reasons is denial for intrapsychic reasons. This is denial used as a defense to decrease anxiety. When resources for coping are limited and people feel in danger of being overwhelmed, they may resort to this more primitive defense. For them; the possibility of death is too much to face; it just is not happening.

If there is a continuum of intrapsychic to interpersonal denial, then people will fall at different points along the way. Some will be firmly at the intrapsychic position, and others will be focused on the interpersonal dimension. Most may be at some point in between. Many need some time to muster the adaptive coping abilities needed to more squarely face their deaths. Those who are closer to the interpersonal position may need some help to overcome their fears or beliefs. Clinicians who see patients as being in denial are challenged by whether they should intervene psychosocially.

Conventional therapeutic wisdom says one should not interfere with someone's use of a defense. It seems accurate to say that someone who is marginally coping and needs to use denial to survive emotionally should be left to his or her use of denial with only supportive interventions. Those whose denial is rooted in their interpersonal lives often respond well to psychosocial interventions that help to open channels of communication.

INTERVENTION

Psychosocial intervention with a dying patient who appears to be using denial can be fraught with difficulties. The clinician has to be exquisitely sensitive to how the patient is coping with the illness and to his or her changing emotional needs. What is needed is the ability to pace intervention to the patient's readiness to face reality.

It is usually best to find out what a patient believes about the illness. If the patient is convinced that he or she is not dying in spite of being told the facts, trying to convince him or her otherwise would be countertherapeutic. As in any therapeutic relationship, it is necessary to form a relationship first and to develop trust. With time, it may be possible to assess whether their refusal to deal with reality is based on their limited coping resources or their fears of abandonment.

For patients described as intrapsychic deniers, it is best to avoid interventions directed at helping them face the reality of their dying. Supportive interventions that bolster their defenses are best. For those whose denial is more interpersonal, interventions that lead to increased communication with those they love are best. For those who are not yet ready to face reality but who have the ability to cope, it may be best to both bolster their defenses while gradually helping them to face reality.

One of the beliefs attendant to being seriously ill is that one has to maintain a positive attitude at all times or face a worsening of one's condition. Although positive thinking can help in the recovery process, it can pose dangers for someone who is terminally ill. Underlying this belief is the unspoken notion that if you can affect the outcome of your illness then perhaps you were part of what caused it in the first place. This can lead to feelings of guilt and self-blame for not being strong enough to overcome the illness. It is also a way in which people may distance themselves from a dying person's feelings. They may not want to have to deal with the sadness of facing the fact that the person is dying, so they tell the person not to talk "that way" or admonish them if they want to talk about painful feelings. When people tell the dying person not to feel the way they feel or to talk about their fears, it is a fundamental discounting of them as a person. Lazarus (1985) referred to this as trivializing the distress of the dying person.

The following case shows how it can be possible to maintain hope while facing the reality of death.

CASE ILLUSTRATION

John

John was a 38-year-old engineer with two young daughters who was dying of metastatic melanoma. He had taken a year off with his family to sail around the

Caribbean. In the past year, he had been back and was working on an important breakthrough in his field. Once diagnosed, he joined a wellness group and started treatment. He was certain that he would beat the disease.

He was referred to hospice after his wife reported that he was too weak to get out of bed. At the hospice intake session, he said that he was certain that he would not die and just needed to regain his strength. His wife was realistic and needed a lot of support. She was concerned about her two daughters, who were very close to John, and how they would react to his death. Her mother had just arrived to help but was still grieving over the death of her husband less than a year earlier.

We agreed that the best approach was to continue to support John's hope but to gradually work on his ability to face the current reality. In conversations with John, it became apparent that he was single-mindedly focused on the wellness philosophy. He believed that if his will were strong enough, he could beat the cancer. To help him with this, we enlisted the aid of his wellness group's facilitator. She was a marriage and family counselor who was quite cooperative and understanding about the situation.

John placed a great deal of faith in her, and when she came to say that the end was near and that he had done all that was possible to help in his healing, he was able to begin facing the possibility of his death. We continued to support John's need for hope but helped him to allow for the possibility that he could die soon. We appealed to his paternal side to encourage him to talk with his daughters about his life and the possibility that he might not always be there.

John never regained his strength, nor was he able to deal with his painful guilt over having triggered his disease during the boat trip. He had ignored the changes in his skin that preceded the diagnosis. He did remain comfortable up to the end and died at home with his family. His young daughters were able to say good-bye to him before he died and helped with his care. His wife and mother-in-law received emotional and bereavement support and were able to help each other. This case illustrates the importance of meeting a person where the person is in his or her readiness to hear painful information and then pacing psychosocial intervention to the person's willingness to face reality.

From denial, I now turn to the important issue of euthanasia. In the next chapter, hospices' role in the debate over the right to die is explored.

Chapter Ten

A Right to Die?

Euthanasia is currently one of the most hotly debated topics of our time. A growing number of states in the United States have held referendums on whether physicians should be allowed to provide terminally ill patients with the means to die. State legislatures have attempted to make physician-assisted suicide (PAS) a distinctly illegal act. U.S. courts have tended to oppose laws banning suicide and in some federal districts (2nd and 9th) have recognized a right to suicide.

In the Ninth Circuit case *Washington v. Glucksberg* (1997 WL 348094, 65 USLW 4669), the court challenged Washington state's ban on assisted suicide asserting that there is a liberty interest protected by our Constitution that protects the right of a mentally competent terminally ill adult to choose PAS. They argued that citizens should be able to control the time and manner of their death.

In the Second Circuit case *Vacco v. Quill* (1997 WL 348037, 65 USLW 4695), the court reviewed a decision that struck down New York's statute prohibiting assisted suicide on the basis that it violated Constitutional guarantees of equal protection. The Second Circuit argued that there was no difference between a terminally ill person who had a legal right to withdraw or forego life support and a gravely ill person seeking to hasten death by suicide.

The Supreme Court overturned both of these decisions and ruled that there is no Constitutional right to assisted suicide. In the Washington case, it cited the enduring themes of our philosophical, legal, and cultural heritage, and the state's rational interest in preserving life, preventing suicide, protecting vulnerable people, protecting the integrity of the medical profession, and protecting family members. In the Vacco case, it noted that there is a fundamental distinction between withdrawing life support and affirmative acts that cause death.

Physicians in the Netherlands have had the ability to assist patients to die for years. Although not completely legal, physicians are allowed to end patients' lives if they follow prescribed guidelines, including patient consent and receipt of a second physician's opinion. Recently, concern has been expressed that these guidelines are ignored with no consequences to the physician.

In the United States, there has been a quiet but not uncommon practice in the medical profession of "medicating the patient out." Some physicians have practiced euthanasia this way for years in private without any safeguards. Recent U.S. reports on medical professionals' involvement in acts that have terminated life have revealed that a large percentage of registered nurses have participated in or had knowledge of patients being euthanized by their physicians. This has invariably been done in an effort to relieve the patient's, or often the family's, distress.

There is also a vocal and polarized argument between those who oppose any form of euthanasia and those who seek to legalize it. Most vocal is pathologist Jack Kevorkian, who has made it his mission to provide people with the means to die. He is supported by public interest groups and by a large percentage of the general public in the United States. Though he has been charged with murder in the deaths of patients who have sought his help in dying, he has been acquitted each time. Public support for PAS may stem from the health care system's difficulty in managing death.

On the other side of this debate are groups that argue for the sanctity of all human life. These groups are often aligned with religious organizations and the anti-abortion movement. They argue that any liberalization of current restrictions on euthanasia will lead to further and further pressures for patients to die. They pose a "slippery slope" argument that once laws and restrictions begin to be relaxed, pressure will build to eliminate all restrictions on euthanasia.

Ethicists take a variety of positions in this debate. It is well recognized that if death results from a physician's efforts to control pain or other symptoms, it is not PAS. However, giving a lethal dose that is far more than needed to control symptoms is PAS. The key issue here is intent. It is also now well established that patients or their surrogates have a right to refuse or withdraw from treatment, including those that can continue life, such as ventilatory support or artificially provided fluid and nutrition.

The fundamental arguments regarding PAS involve one's basic ethical position. Some take the deontological or moralistic position that PAS is fundamentally wrong. Others take a more pragmatic position that one must weigh the benefits and burdens of the situation to find what is right for the patient facing death. These are different basic positions that are hard to reconcile.

What has been notably absent in this debate is the role of hospice care. Hospices offer a middle ground in this argument. Instead of premature death, hospice offers relief from the symptoms and conditions that drive terminally ill people to consider suicide.

THE HOSPICE SOLUTION

The desire for euthanasia is fueled by fear, fear of actual or imagined distress. Those with terminal illnesses, and some with painful chronic illnesses, consider suicide to escape unbearable distress. When that distress is relieved, thoughts of suicide usually recede. Pain is a common distress feared by seriously ill persons. Because hospices are adept at controlling pain, the memory and fear of pain recede with good control.

Of course, there are many other types of distress associated with dying. Besides other physical symptoms, there is distress at being dependent on others for care, unresolved relationships with others, fear of losing control, loss of dignity, and fear of oblivion, to name a few. Hospice as an interdisciplinary system of care looks to address any source of distress in patients and their families.

Being dependent on others can be as much a blessing as a curse. Hospices often redefine the opportunity for family members to care for a patient as an opportunity to give back to someone. Our parents cared for us when we were young, now we can care for them. Our spouse has been our lifelong partner, and providing care is a way of giving thanks as well as a helpful memory during the grieving process.

The opportunity to resolve hurt relationships is one of the most powerful reasons to avoid premature death. Hospice workers often help to heal these relationships before a person dies. Reminding family members that this may be their last opportunity to say "I'm sorry" or "I love you" often gives them permission to make things right. The best death is one that leaves relationships whole.

Modern life is full of anxiety. People try to handle it by attempting to control events. When a terminal illness strikes, one cannot control the outcome. Richard Lazarus (1966) defined the difference between problem- and emotion-focused coping. Problem-focused coping is what people do when there is a problem that needs to be solved: the car breaks down or one has to figure out how to beat a competitor. When faced with a terminal illness, people often try to use problem-focused coping but get frustrated when it does not work and feel helpless.

What they then do is turn to emotion-focused coping. They mediate their internal reactions and adapt to the situation. Some of these reactions are more adaptive than others. Hospice workers help people to understand they are facing a loss of control and to find other things they can realistically control.

Some people hate the idea of losing their independence, having their body image change, or losing roles that are important to their self-esteem. There is not a great deal that anyone can do about these losses except to help them to grieve and come to some accommodation to a new reality.

The impending loss of the self and fear of the unknown is also difficult to address. For those with a belief system that includes a continued existence after death, there is usually less anxiety, and spiritual support helps them to overcome their doubts. For those who have resolved themselves that there is no afterlife, there may be less anxiety. Those who are unsure (agnostic) are most likely to be in conflict over the impending oblivion.

An additional problem for those facing death is the likelihood that clinical depression will color attitudes and decisions about continuing life. Faced with the stereotype that death is always painful and full of indignity and being vulnerable to depression at feeling helpless, many contemplate suicide as a way out.

Rather than encouraging a hasty end to life, it makes more sense to find out what the source of distress is and then respond to it. It would be very unusual for a dying person to want euthanasia when his or her symptoms are controlled, he or she is not depressed, and he or she feels supported by those around them. This is exactly what hospices strive for in the care of their patients.

UNBEARABLE SUFFERING

There are a small number of patients whose suffering cannot be controlled without impairment of consciousness. This may be due to severe neuropathic pain, extreme disfigurement, or circumstances that cannot be resolved. For patients with pain that cannot be controlled without impairment of consciousness, the prevailing opinion is that barbiturate sedation is appropriate. The level of sedation should be enough to produce unconsciousness but not necessarily death. This rarely occurs and is at the final stages of the illness.

All efforts to control pain by other means will have to have been attempted before this. For severe neuropathic pain, this may include use of coanalgesics, very large doses of narcotics, nerve block, and so forth. Sedation is a last resort but will remove perception of pain. The patient would not be expected to regain consciousness, and death would be expected usually within days, depending on the patient's condition.

Other rare situations where patients are faced with potentially unbearable circumstances include extreme disfigurement. This can include patients with large fungating lesions, head and neck tumors growing out of orifices, and widespread Kaposi's sarcoma. In these cases, efforts are made to control problems with sight and odor. Bandaging and use of chlorophyll or charcoal may help.

Suffering is a subjective experience. What constitutes suffering for one may be easily tolerable for another. As with pain, it is whatever the patient perceives it to be. It is often surprising that a patient may be able to cope with something that someone else might find unbearable. What can be taken from this is that there is always something that can be done in situations of extreme suffering that may diminish the patient's desire for euthanasia.

THE PROBLEM WITH EUTHANASIA

Euthanasia is, in this context, the taking of life. Treatment accurately aimed at relieving symptoms that results in death is not euthanasia. Neither is the withdrawal of artificial life support or treatments that postpone a death that would otherwise occur naturally. Either the physician or another takes the patient's life or the patient takes his or her own life by suicide. This does not constitute murder, as it has been requested by the patient.

As previously discussed, it is much more effective to deal with the fears and problems that drive the patient to want an early death than it is to provide the patient with the means to suicide. The decision to seek euthanasia is a complex one. Decisions are often colored by interpersonal dynamics. Patients may feel compelled to seek the end to relieve the burden they feel they have become on their family.

Hospice care can help relieve this burden in most cases. There are some families, however, who are ill prepared to cope and need more than can be provided even through hospice. In these situations, alternate caregiving arrangements need to be made to provide for the patient's needs either through privately hired in-home care or a residential or nursing care facility.

A recent documentary in the Netherlands intended to show the positive side of the Dutch euthanasia policy. In the film, a terminally ill patient was interviewed. During the interview, the patient hardly spoke. His wife did all the talking and conveyed how difficult his illness had been. The patient consented to euthanasia, but it was clear from the couple interaction that he was anything but a willing subject. In spite of a belief in the primacy of patient autonomy, health care workers forget how much all health care decisions are made in the context of a family system.

Patients make their treatment decisions with the family's reactions in mind. A treatment that the patient does not want will be accepted because the family wants the patient to fight. The patient does not want to disappoint loved ones. If treatment is refused, the family may feel the patient wants to end his or her life because he or she does not love them and would just as soon be dead. In the same way, patients may come to believe the family is tired of caring for them or that everyone would be better off if they were gone.

In addition to family, health care providers and society exert subtle or overt pressure on patients to consent to excessive disease-oriented therapy. Other patients may be similarly pressured to consent to euthanasia if it is legalized. These unspoken dynamics are very powerful and can greatly influence decisions about euthanasia.

Other problems with euthanasia include determining who is terminally ill, who will administer fatal doses, where does one draw the line, and the problem of clinical depression. At present, it is rather difficult to determine how long anyone will live. The SUPPORT Investigators (1995) study previously mentioned developed a complex algorithm for determining probability of death for patients grouped with seven types of terminal conditions. One of the study authors, Joanne Lynn, commented that any method for determining prognosis that had a .50 or greater probability of accuracy was probably as good as one can get at this time.

The NHO has had a task force working on the problem of determining prognosis in terminally ill patients since 1994. Guidelines have been developed that can help in identifying patients who are likely to die within 6 months. These guidelines are based on what is found in the current literature. Probably the best that can be said about their accuracy is that they are not wrong.

As there is no hard science to determine when someone is terminally ill, how is a person to decide if he or she qualifies for the proposed PAS? Current referendum efforts limit euthanasia to those who are terminally ill. Many of the patients seen by Jack Kevorkian are not terminally ill. They may have an incurable condition that causes them distress, but they are not terminally ill by the usual current definition of less than 6 months of life if the illness runs its normal course. So should the definition be expanded to all who have chronic illnesses? This could open a floodgate of potential patients who may request or be pressured to accept PAS.

Many patients who request PAS are too debilitated to actually take a lethal dose. They must have someone's help to accomplish termination of life. This poses a dilemma. Physicians often do not want to administer death. It is fairly easy to write a prescription to give to a patient. It is much harder to give the lethal dose. Family members have the same problem. They do not want to have the memory of actually being responsible for ending their loved one's life. So who will provide assistance in the act of ending the patient's life?

I have said that the boundary of terminal illness is vague. So where does one draw the line? A recent report from the Netherlands (Pijnenborg, van der Maas, van Delden, & Looman, 1993) showed that there have been a growing number of cases of involuntary euthanasia (0.8% of all deaths). This number may be much lower than actual due to underreporting. In these cases, the physician has determined without consent that the patient's life should be ended. The physician may believe that the patient is suffering and it would be the humane thing to do. Physicians are supposed to get another physician's assent but often this is done by another colleague who has never seen the patient.

What is troubling about these cases is their frequency and the lack of any oversight. In 1990, based on an anonymous physician survey, approximately 1,000 people received involuntary euthanasia in the Netherlands. In 41% of these cases, the physician had no information on the patient's wishes. Although the fears of those who use the slippery slope argument may be exaggerated, there is serious cause for concern that making euthanasia available will lead to abuses. In addition, it has been reported that as many as 25% of those undergoing PAS in the Netherlands are initially unsuccessful (Hendin, Rutenfrancs, & Zylich, 1997). This raises the spectre of a painful dysphoric lingering death rather than the smooth transition sought by patients.

One of the symptoms of clinical depression is a tendency toward suicidal ideation, and depressed people are more apt to commit suicide. When depression is properly treated, suicidal tendencies are diminished. Terminally and chronically ill people are vulnerable to clinical depression, which often goes untreated. Some assume that the illness is cause to be depressed and that treatment is unnecessary.

This goes back to the old exogenous versus endogenous distinction in depression. It used to be assumed that depression caused by external factors (exogenous) did not respond to treatment, whereas internally produced depression (endogenous) did. Nowadays this distinction is no longer considered relevant, though those with vegetative signs of depression (psychomotor retardation, sleep disturbance, etc.) tend to respond better to antidepressant therapy.

There is real danger in allowing depressed patients to go through with suicide without treatment. The same is true for all other treatable forms of distress. Rather than ending life, it makes more sense to treat the underlying cause of the distress.

SOCIETY'S ROLE

Recent polls have shown that the majority of Americans favor legalizing PAS. This opinion seems to derive from the collective social belief that people ought to have as much freedom as possible and that the government is interfering in our lives too much. The courts have supported this position by declaring laws against PAS unconstitutional.

Attempts to legalize PAS in the United States have not fared well. The first to pass on referendum in Oregon was declared unconstitutional by the court. Many other states are experimenting with the legalization of PAS. At this writing, it appears that both efforts to legalize PAS and efforts to make it illegal are failing. This leaves an ambiguous gray area—which is possibly where PAS is best left.

Many national organizations have expressed strong opposition to PAS. The American Medical Association along with the NHO have declared strong opposition to PAS. NHO has asked hospices to serve all terminally ill patients, even those who desire euthanasia.

Should PAS be legalized and recognized, hospices would be put in a particularly difficult position. Should any of their patients wish to avail themselves of PAS, the hospice would find itself in a dilemma. Would they support patients in ending their lives in the manner they choose, or would they try to dissuade them? Certainly all hospices would want to address any treatable distress so the patient would have no reason for PAS. If, however, the patient still insisted on PAS, what would the hospice do?

Some hospice programs are addressing the issue proactively. A few have taken the position that they would discharge the patient from the hospice. They take the position that this is like the patient who insists on receiving curative treatment and leaves hospice. Hospice neither hastens nor postpones death. It also seems like abandoning the patient at a crucial moment. Patients may chose to leave hospice but to discharge the patient does not seem therapeutic. Yet what is a hospice to do if it is adamantly opposed to PAS?

Other programs support the philosophical position that patient choice is the most important value in this discussion. Even if they oppose PAS, they support the patient's right to decide for him- or herself. If the hospice decides it will continue to serve the patient who insists on PAS, then comes the difficult decision regarding what role hospice will play. Should they actively assist the patient in arranging PAS? Can they stand back and allow PAS to go forward without any role?

As with any ethical dilemma, there are few hard-and-fast rules. Each case may have to be addressed in a dialogue with the patient and family. Hospice will have to negotiate its role in PAS with the same sensitivity it handles other difficult psychosocial issues. What is right for one patient may not work for another.

CASE ILLUSTRATION

Dr. K.

Dr. K. was one of the early leaders in the hospice community. He was a founding medical director of a hospice and a strong proponent of symptom control and hospice care. Over the years, he became more cynical about hospice's ability to relieve distress. When his wife died following a stroke precipitated from a simple surgery, he became quite bitter about health care in general. He was depressed and wished his life would end. He had long been a proponent of legalizing euthanasia.

About 18 months after his wife's lingering death, Dr. K. was diagnosed with widely metastatic cancer with an unknown primary. His surgeon did an open-and-close laparotomy. He advised Dr. K. to get his affairs in order. A few months before this, Dr. K. had fallen in love again and was living with his girlfriend. After returning home, he was referred to hospice. During the hospice intake discussion, he said, "The moment my pain is too uncomfortable, I plan to kill myself, and if you have a problem with that, leave right now."

Hospice services were initiated, and Dr. K. insisted on being in control. Over the course of his last 6 weeks, hospice staff provided nursing, emotional, and spiritual support. He decided to marry his girlfriend, and the hospice chaplain performed the service in his home. Equipment was brought in and medication provided. Family were taught how to provide care. A full bottle of sleeping pills remained in the headboard of his bed. In one conversation, he stated his desire to make his death a statement for euthanasia by writing an article about his suicide and publishing it posthumously. His main worry was for his wife and the possibility of getting his family in legal trouble if they were to help him end his life.

In the following days, he continued to decline but remained comfortable. As his death neared, those close to him gathered around him. The day before his death, I visited and said my good-bye. He was unable to speak, but he held my hand and smiled. The full bottle of pills lay nearby. Somehow I knew he never reached the point where his distress was bad enough for him to end his own life.

This completes the section on pitfalls. In the next chapter, the unique aspects of hospice care are explored.

RECOMMENDED READING

Hastings Center. (1987). *Guidelines on the termination of life sustaining treatment and the care of the dying.* New York: The Hastings Center.

Jonson, A., Seigler, M., & Winslade, W. (1982). *Clinical ethics: A practical approach to ethical decisions in clinical medicine.* New York: Macmillan.

Morgan, J. D. (1996). *Ethical issues in the care of the dying and bereaved aged.* Amityville, NY: Baywood.

Winslade, W., & Ross, J. W. (1986). *Choosing life or death: A guide for patients, families, and professionals.* New York: Free Press.

Part Three

Promise

In this section, the reader will explore some issues for the future of the hospice movement. Areas covered include unique aspects of hospice care, outcome measurement, and issues the movement must face in the years ahead.

Chapter 11

Why Hospice Is Unique in the Health Care System

"A life is not important except in its impact on other lives."

—Mrs. Jackie Robinson

Most view hospice as just another health care provider that is not particularly unique. The individual services provided can by and large be found outside of hospice. Most dying patients are cared for by other providers throughout the health care system. So why do those associated with hospices consider hospice care to be unique?

TRUE TEAMWORK

This book has discussed types of team functioning and hospices' interdisciplinary approach. When this works at its best, it is a remarkable process. Team meetings enhance a sense of community within hospice. Each member of the team is valued as an essential contributor to the process of reaching a good death.

In many multidisciplinary health care teams, the physician dominates the discussion and there is clearly a hierarchical structure. The contributions of those higher up in the hierarchy are given greater value and credence. When the hospice interdisciplinary team is working well, there is no hierarchy. Each team member's contribution is valued on the basis of its relevance to understanding the unique process the patient and family are facing.

At another level, the hospice team functioning is a kind of support group for those faced with caring for dying patients. They are able to share the joys and sorrows experienced in day-to-day care. When they are wrestling with a difficult problem, they can go to the brain trust of the team and help find a solution. The rest of the team serves as a witness to the work of each team member. A nurse can describe how the dying process went and be acknowledged for the patient's having a good death. If things did not go well, the team can help to gain perspective on how this came to pass.

Interaction in hospice team meetings is collaborative. The primary aim is to develop a team sense of who the patient and family are and how they can best be served by hospice. In a typical team meeting, new admissions are discussed in detail. A medical history is given by the nurse case manager, followed by a psychosocial and spiritual assessment from the social worker and chaplain. Current problems are identified, and plans for intervention are developed.

At these meetings, there is also discussion of deaths since the last meeting, problem cases, and any updates on stable patients. The flavor of discussion is planning for the best care and coordination of who will take the lead in meeting particular needs. Each member of the team is acknowledged and valued for his or her contribution. This is not to say that people are not challenged. There can be spirited discussion of important issues of how best to provide care as well as identification of problems that require policy or practice changes in the agency.

PREVENTION

Hospice's effectiveness in controlling the distress of those who are terminally ill is directly related to its focus on prevention. Any symptom is easier to manage if you prevent it from happening in the first place. Using pain as an example, say hospice admits a patient whose pain is out of control. The experience operates as reinforcing feedback. The more the pain remains out of control, the less confidence the patient has that his or her pain can be controlled.

Through aggressive palliative care, hospice is able to control the patient's pain, usually within a short period of time. Medication is dosed so that the level of analgesic in the blood is high enough to prevent the pain's return. After a while, the memory and fear of the pain is diminished so much so that less medication may be needed. The same approach works with other symptoms as well.

Hospices know where the pitfalls are when facing death. After working with so many people who have died, hospice professionals develop a sense of the common psychosocial challenges facing the dying. Each dying person faces these challenges in a different way. Hospice caregivers help patients and their families to face difficult decisions about care. They educate about the different treatments available and the benefits and burdens of each. Hospice team members help the patient formulate goals for care at the end of life. These goals will determine how the patient is treated. Areas addressed include use of antibiotics, blood transfusions, oxygen, respirators, cardiopulmonary resuscitation, dialysis, chemotherapy, radiation therapy, ambulance transport, IV therapies, tube feedings, and hospitalization.

Depending on state laws, hospice team members help see that advanced directives and other legal protections are in place to ensure the patient's wishes are obeyed and the patient is protected from unwanted treatment. It is usually appropriate to also help the patient and family make or finalize arrangements for funeral services. Dealing with all these difficult questions ahead of time is definitely a preventative service. When these issues are left unresolved, there can be a great deal of turmoil in the family about what to do. When plans are made, everyone can relax more by knowing what the patient wants.

DEINSTITUTIONALIZATION

Over the past 50 years, health care has been delivered more and more in institutional settings. Following World War II, there was a major push to ensure that hospitals were available to all citizens in the United States. These hospitals became the center point for delivery of health care. As medical technology advanced, so too did the services based in hospitals. As the population has aged and hospitals have had to specialize in the care of the sickest patients, the nursing home industry has developed into an enormous institution for the ongoing care of elderly and disabled persons.

As a society, people have come to both love and fear these institutions. They insist that acute care services be immediately available for any illness and demand that these services be effective in handling all medical problems. When a medical problem cannot be solved, the institution often continues to make the attempt and the patient must endure a juggernaut of treatments, tests, and procedures.

When all these efforts fail, the patient is either left to die in a sterile hospital environment or is transferred to the nursing facility, there to wait out a death sentence while being cared for by strangers. All people have strong feelings about spending their last days helpless, in the hands of overworked and underpaid caregivers. There are, of course, some excellent nursing facilities and hospitals where staff are very caring and allow patients to express their unique humanity. The point is that they are still institutions where one is a patient and must conform to the environment. They are not one's home where the person is ultimately in control, surrounded by the memories and collection of a lifetime. In one's home, you can listen to the music you like, you can get that book you want, you can decide what to eat and when to eat it. You can laugh or cry or belch without fear of upsetting the next person.

So it is no wonder that there has been a gradual rebellion against the institutionalization of health care. The hospice movement is in fact part of a consumer's movement. People do not want health care at the convenience of health care providers. They want care that is directed to their needs as an individual. They want care that allows them to remain as independent and human as possible. They want care that is provided where they live. If they have to be cared for in a facility, they want few rules and to be treated as individuals. It is not surprising that one of the first things Dr. Saunders envisioned at St. Christopher's Hospice was a different set of house rules for her patients. There would be 24-hour-a-day visiting. Patients would be allowed to bring their own things into the room to make it more homelike. Children would be allowed and encouraged to visit. Patients would always be treated with kindness, respect, and courtesy. There would be a large number of staff to care for the patients. The afternoon tea tray would be brought around.

In the United States' inpatient hospices, the same philosophy pervades. There are some lovely freestanding hospice facilities where patients are cared for. They get food when they want it, served by family or to family. Accommodations are provided for family to sleep over in the patient's room. There may be a sound system and videotapes. Rooms are decorated to be more homelike. Patients will get their bath when they prefer it. Length of stay will be determined by how well their symptoms are managed rather than their DRG or diagnosis.

Care in the acute hospital setting has become enormously expensive. Care in the home has emerged as a much more cost-effective alternative. It makes more sense to use some resources to maintain a patient at home than to have to spend a lot to provide for all their needs in a facility. Once patients enter a health care facility, they are the responsibility of the institution. Extended family are moved aside and discouraged from taking responsibility. Sure, they are encouraged to visit, but they are usually not allowed to deliver any care. This is not the case in hospice facilities, where active involvement in delivering care is strongly encouraged and is critical in training the family to continue meeting the patient's care needs at home.

Home health care is provided by a number of providers in the United States. Home health agencies, homemaker services, home infusion companies, durable medical equipment providers, and private duty nursing pools all provide services to patients at home. They most often deliver care to patients who are recovering from an illness and help rehabilitate them to the point where they are able to care for themselves. They also provide health services in the home to chronically ill patients whose prognosis is uncertain. These patients may use home health care to be able to leave the hospital early or to prevent readmission. Home health agencies also care for terminally ill patients but are less effective at meeting their total needs than hospice programs.

In the United States, home health care has not been set up to effectively prevent hospitalization and institutionalization. When the patient is in a crisis, home health agencies must contact the physician, who routinely has the patient sent to a hospital emergency room. From there, the patient is usually given an extensive diagnostic workup and is admitted. In many parts of the United States, the home health service is not available 24 hours a day, and patients in crisis must seek out an emergency room themselves.

In contrast, hospices usually plan ahead for these crises. Orders are given ahead of time for managing exacerbations. Medical staff are always available 24 hours a day to go to the home if necessary. The emergency room is routinely avoided. If admission is needed, a direct admission is arranged. As the goals of care are agreed on, there are no true emergencies in the usual sense. The goal is management of the symptoms. Anything that can be done in the hospital for a hospice patient can be done in the home as well.

Hospice's success in keeping patients at home and out of institutions is due in large part to its focus on family involvement in caregiving. The patient's attachment network (family) actually does the largest share of the patient care. The simple secret is that families usually require only permission to do what is necessary to keep the patient at home. Health care providers sometimes prefer to keep family caregivers in the dark about how to take care of the patient. This may be done out of a misguided concern that they might harm the patient or as a way of ensuring their own job security.

Whatever the motive, there is every reason to teach families as much as possible about caregiving. Their education must always be tempered by an understanding of each individual's capacity for learning as well as his or her emotional history with the patient. Nonetheless, hospices have found that even families with limited capabilities are able to do a great deal of nursing care. It requires giving them permission to care so often denied when the patient is in an institution.

Once families are empowered to provide care, they are usually eager to learn the specifics of how to transfer, feed, toilet, do mouth care and skin care, and give medication to their family member. This does great things to alleviate feelings of helplessness and anxiety and helps ease the grief process. It also makes the difference between being able to be cared for at home rather than in an institution.

HOSPICE WORKERS

Is there something unique about the people who work in hospices or are they just like other health care providers? For the most part, they are like other health care workers, except they too have been given permission to act in a different way toward their patients. The tradition of hospice caregiving calls them to bring their whole self to the work they do. Some of this difference can be heard in the words of the patients and families served by hospices. Over and over, they say things like "There is no way Mom could have died at home without hospice" or "I don't know how I could have done it without you" or "The love and caring I received was overwhelming, we thank you with all our hearts, we will never forget what you did for us, you all are part of our family now."

Why is it that hospices receive such accolades from those they serve? It is likely because of the dedication of the staff and volunteers who view their work as more than a job. Hospices certainly have their share of difficult employees, but the kind of person who chooses to work in a hospice is seeking to express more than just a set of job skills. Most have had many years of experience in the health care field and have been frustrated in not being allowed to express true caring.

Health care workers usually have a vision of what it is like to be a caregiver. This vision goes something like this: I will help people who are in real need to be comforted or cured and will feel satisfied that my efforts make a real difference in the lives of people I come to care about. After working in a health care institution, these workers come to experience a different reality: I am over-whelmed by the needs of so many whom I can neither help or get to know as people. Nurses spend their time running from IV to IV, and social workers spend their time handling paperwork without ever getting to do the counseling they expected to do.

Work in hospice offers these idealists an opportunity to do what they came into health care to do. They actually get to help people and get to make a difference that they can see. This may be an oversimplification, but it works. Hospices encourage staff and volunteers to get to know their patients and to become somewhat involved with them emotionally. This involvement does carry risks, but the rewards can be worth it.

Dr. Dale Larson (1993), a psychologist from Santa Clara University who trains hospice workers, has described the concept *accurate empathy* to demon-strate how hospice workers can be effective in helping without burning out. Imagine a continuum on which one end is the caregiver who is totally empathetic. This caregiver is so involved with the dying patient and family that she or he moves in and becomes part of the family. This is a very painful place to be and cannot be done very long. On the other end is the detached professional who keeps a professional distance and never gets involved with a patient. This person does not get much satisfaction from the work and feels bad about him- or herself.

Hospice workers tend to start out as the hot empathetic person who bonds with the patient and family. After experiencing a deep sense of loss when patients die, they tend to pull away from getting so close to protect themselves. This leaves them feeling cold and unsatisfied, so they go back to the close hot end of the continuum. After a while they begin to feel like a yo-yo and cannot be very effective.

To survive in hospice work, one must first have a strong sense of empathy for the patient. One learns that if you get too involved you become ineffective. So good hospice caregivers find a balance where they are able to show their caring without becoming too invested or enmeshed emotionally with those they care for.

This healthy caring is one of the things that families find special about hospice. They are used to cold impersonal caregivers and may feel burdened by those who want to get too close or do everything for them. Caregivers who lift the family up by encouraging their involvement in patient care and praising the work they do are most appreciated.

PSYCHOSOCIAL AND SPIRITUAL CARE

When hospice care is suggested, it is often because it is believed that hospice can provide more emotional and spiritual support than can be found elsewhere. This is true. Health care is still quite segmented. Mental health services are segregated from medical care, and spiritual care is really not considered part of the health care system at all. Hospices are the only providers that have integrated these components into a comprehensive program. Psychological care and social support are integral parts of hospice services. Chaplaincy and spiritual support are part of the assessment and caregiving process in any hospice. The bereavement follow-up services provided by hospices are also unique.

Psychosocial services can only be paid for in the health care system if the person has a mental disorder. In hospice this is unnecessary, as all patients and families are eligible to receive counseling. Their circumstances qualify them to receive this care. Good hospice programs provide as much counseling as requested and needed. Every patient and family ordinarily has a social worker assigned to visit as needed to help everyone prepare emotionally for the impending loss. There is usually a crisis response at the time of death to increase the amount of psychosocial support provided.

The provision of spiritual or pastoral care is a neglected part of the health care continuum. Beyond providing chaplains to visit patients while in the hospital, there are no pastoral care services in health care. In hospice, a significant amount of attention is given to ensuring that patients receive the spiritual support they need. Most hospices have chaplaincy staff who are available to visit patients at home, and all are required to address spiritual needs through coordination with community clergy. Including spiritual or transcendent needs in the hospice plan of care is essential to having a truly interdisciplinary program. Addressing these needs is critical to achieving quality of life for many dying patients. Spiritual care is for many patients the most important aspect of care, as it is focused on their most important fears and opportunities for growth.

The provision of bereavement services may be the most unique aspect of hospice care. No other provider has established an in-depth response to the needs of grieving people. The mental health system considers bereavement a legitimate focus of treatment but has done little to develop services for the bereaved as bereavement is not considered a disorder and therefore is not reimbursable. Hospices are in the forefront of creating services specifically designed for populations of grieving people.

BEYOND SYMPTOM MANAGEMENT

Most people view the experience of facing death as an unpleasant reality in which the best one can hope for is the absence of pain and distress. Hospice workers have discovered after many years of caring for those near death that there is also the possibility that the end of life can be a time of growth and positive feelings.

Many dying patients have reported that as death approached, a number of opportunities are presented. They are confronted with a finite measure of remaining life, and this can bring about a focusing of the mind. A change in perspective occurs such that unimportant issues are ignored and things that matter to the patient take the foreground.

This is only possible if the symptoms of the terminal illness are controlled. Without relief from pain or other distressing physical symptoms, the patient cannot attend to other concerns. Once freed from physical distress, the patient is able to attend to psychological, emotional, interpersonal, social, and transcendent or spiritual matters.

DEVELOPMENTAL LANDMARKS AND TASKS FOR THE END OF LIFE

One of the foremost proponents for the view that the end of life holds opportunities for growth is Ira Byock. Byock has lectured widely and written about these opportunities to international audiences. A hospice physician since 1978, he has learned what he knows of this from the experiences shared by many of his dying patients. Byock has developed a working typology for helping people understand these opportunities for growth.

Byock (1997) promoted the notion of "dying well," the desired outcome for those facing death. By this he meant a continuation of the lifelong developmental process. This process continues during the time of approaching death and actually may accelerate. Byock's 10 major developmental landmarks and tasks include the following.

Sense of completion with worldly affairs: Transfer of fiscal, legal, and formal social responsibilities

The patient gets his or her affairs in order. A will is done, funeral arrangements are made, and social responsibilities are terminated.

Sense of completion in relationships with community: Closure of multiple social relationships (employment, commerce, organizational, and congregational)

Components include expressions of regret, expressions of forgiveness, acceptance, gratitude, and appreciation—leave taking, the saying of good-bye. This task involves the advance transfer of any business responsibilities to others. It may mean arranging for a family member to take over running the business or liquidation of partnerships. One may have to resign from organizations or discontinue attendance at meetings. As illness progresses, attendance at church or synagogue is disrupted; it is hoped that the clergy is available to continue providing support.

Along with this process of withdrawal, there are many opportunities to share regret at being unable to continue. There is also often an outpouring of support and gratitude to be received. The process of leaving can be a time of acknowledgment from others that might not otherwise occur.

Sense of meaning about one's individual life:
Life review—the telling of one's stories;
transmission of knowledge and wisdom

The opportunity to review one's life before death is a transformative process. The process of stepping out of your life to review it can have a profound effect. Every life has some important milestones and major events. These can be as basic as the birth of children, service in the community or military, or career or of considerable significance, such as heroic action, invention, or other creative activity.

Hospice workers often recommend a review of one's life as a therapeutic activity with persons facing death. When written or taped, it can be suggested as a gift to the family who are left behind. This oral life history includes many stories from the person's life. In addition to recounting the important milestones in one's life, it is an opportunity to convey a person's philosophy about life and one's personal wisdom about life. It is especially helpful for a person with young children to leave this as a legacy to live on in the lives of those left behind.

Experienced love of self:
Self-acknowledgment and self-forgiveness

Often people are their own worst enemies and harshest critics. The time before dying can be an opportunity (perhaps for the first time) to genuinely appreciate oneself and to forgive oneself for those things one regrets doing.

Experienced love of others:
Acceptance of worthiness

For those with poor self-esteem, the admiration and love of others is always sought but rarely embraced. Most of us feel unworthy at times. As death approaches, people may allow themselves to feel the love others have for them.

Sense of completion in relationships with family and friends: Reconciliation, fullness of communication, and closure in each of one's important relationships

Component tasks include expression of regret, forgiveness and acceptance, expressions of gratitude and appreciation, acceptance of gratitude and appreciation, expressions of affection, and leave taking; the saying of good-bye.

The opportunity to say good-bye to the people who form one's immediate attachment network can be profoundly moving. In saying good-bye, people allow for the expression of many powerful and healing emotions. Corrective emotional experiences can occur that can transform a lifetime of emotional pain into feelings of relief and release. In the presence of death, people have permission to show emotions and to say things they otherwise would not. This creates the opportunity for closure as well as the possibility of deep feelings of love and well-being.

Acceptance of the finality of life, of one's existence as an individual

This includes acknowledgment of the totality of personal loss represented by one's dying and experience of personal pain of existential loss, expression of the depth of personal tragedy that dying represents, decathexis (emotional withdrawal) from worldly affairs and cathexis (emotional connection) with an enduring construct, and acceptance of dependency

Death is the loss of one's self. Each dying person must face this on a personal level and grieve over what is to be lost. It is at this juncture that people can pull away from life and withdraw. Rather than being a negative retreat, however, it can be a time for feeling connected to whatever enduring construct for continuation one feels.

Sense of a new self (personhood) beyond personal loss

Out of this personal grief process comes a new sense of self that is the essence of personhood. Once a person strips away all that he or she has come to think of as him- or herself (profession, roles, learned behaviors), what is left is that part that has not changed throughout his or her life. This essential unchanging part is truly who one is.

Sense of meaning about life in general

This includes achieving a sense of awe, recognition of a transcendent realm, and developing and achieving a sense of comfort with chaos.

At this point in the developmental process, the dying person has completed saying good-bye, has grieved for the loss of self, and has gotten to the core of him- or herself. From this may come an opportunity to transcend the self and to see life in a different way. Each experience may seem fresh and meaningful. Instead of trying to control life, one may find comfort with the way things are; an understanding that life goes on with or without one and that things will be all right.

Surrender to the transcendent, to the unknown: letting go

So often with those near death, there is a hesitation about leaving life. People hold on to those they love or are not sure of their faith or ready to face the unknown. Hospice workers often have to coach the family to get them to tell the dying person that it is all right to leave, that they will be fine. A final task is being able to let go and to embrace or surrender to whatever is next. It is allowing oneself to step off the precipice and go on.

Dealing with the preceding developmental issues can lead to the possibility that dying may be a time for a heightened sense of well-being. This may not always be a pleasant feeling. The struggle of growth can be painful but leads to a greater sense of mastery and integration.

Rather than only focusing on the negative, problem-oriented aspects of the dying process, clinicians need to be receptive to the possibilities of growth. Even though clinicians are used to being limited in the health care system to only working on problems, hospice care is one of the few examples of a milieu where helping the patient to grow is acceptable.

There is no prohibition from funding sources against including intervention that results in personal growth. Other health care services like medicine and mental health can only receive reimbursement for treating disorders. In hospice, once you have a terminal illness with the requisite prognosis you are entitled to psychosocial and spiritual support that can go beyond the treatment of problems or disorders. This can only be done if the hospice program recognizes this as a legitimate area of concern and need.

Hospice workers should be cautioned that imposing expectations that the dying person should grow during this period can be unhelpful. There is a fine but important line between suggesting possibilities for growth that the person may not have considered and pushing the idea of developmental changes that the patient is neither interested in nor capable of attaining.

It is also important that all areas of suffering be addressed as the person goes through this time. To try to skip emotional pain on the way to developing a transcendent perspective is like trying to ignore physical pain to focus on psychological concerns. The dying person cannot deal with emotional issues with a body aching from bone metastases. Nor can the dying person develop a new sense of self when surrounded by unresolved interpersonal conflicts.

This chapter has examined what differentiates hospice as a health care provider in a general sense. The next chapter examines more specific measures of effectiveness.

Chapter 12

How Good Is Hospice Care?

"Statistics are like a bikini. What they reveal is suggestive but what they conceal is vital."

—Aaron Levenstein

Hospice care may have some unique attributes in the health care system, but is it better than "traditional" or mainstream care of the dying patient? What proof is there that it is as good as its proponents claim? Hospices have not been especially good at collecting data or doing research. Most hospices lack the funding or expertise to carry out research. Even so, some efforts are being made to take a hard look at the care being delivered and its impact on both the patients and families served and the system it affects.

RESULTS OF STUDIES OF HOSPICE EFFECTIVENESS

It is interesting that most studies of hospice effectiveness to date have looked at cost effectiveness rather than clinical outcomes. Cost effectiveness has been a major variable in studies in an effort to preserve funding and expand coverage for hospice care. The results of these studies are equivocal in that some researchers have found no cost savings, and others have noted substantial savings. An early study of hospice care (Kane, Wales, Bernstein, Leibowitz, & Kaplan,

1984) done entirely in the Veterans Administration health care system found no significant difference in treatment costs or satisfaction with care between hospice and conventional care patients. Critics of this study questioned some of the measures used and noted that the intervention (hospice care provided in the Veterans Administration system) may not have been characteristic of care provided by other hospice providers. The study was also done before the implementation of the Hospice Medicare Benefit, which greatly enhanced the services hospices could offer. It was, however, the only large randomized trial to be conducted on hospice versus no-hospice care.

Random assignment (participants are assigned to either a treatment or control group on the basis of a table of random numbers) has been greatly resisted by hospice investigators. There is already a widespread belief in the value and efficacy of hospice care. To deny someone access to this care in order to study its effectiveness is viewed as unethical by some researchers.

A national hospice study was funded by the HCFA to analyze hospices' cost effectiveness. Results revealed that home-care-based hospice programs' treatment costs were lower than the costs of conventional care regardless of length of stay (Mor, Greer, & Kastenbaum, 1988). Hospital-based hospice programs' treatment costs were less than conventional care costs only for patients with lengths of stay in hospice of less than 2 months. Although compelling, there remain questions about whether selection bias may have influenced these results, as randomization was not practicable.

Results of the first 3 years of experience under the Hospice Medicare Benefit have been widely reported. According to Medicare Part A data, $1.26 was saved for every dollar spent on hospice care. However, questions have again been raised about whether these savings are overstated as a result of persistent selection effects (Birenbaum & Kidder, 1992). Were those using hospice less likely to use more expensive services before death or were they perhaps healthier than other dying patients?

In an effort to address some of these selection questions, the NHO commissioned an independent study of the Medicare data tapes (NHO, 1995a). Lewin VH1 analyzed data on 191,545 Medicare recipients who died between July 1 to December 31, 1992. Costs for all services were analyzed during the last 12 months of life. The study included 39,719 recipients who were hospice users. A comparison group of 123,323 patients who did not receive any hospice care was carefully matched for age, sex, and disease. This larger group was matched with the hospice group to determine population differences.

Results of this study demonstrated that on average Medicare beneficiaries with cancer who enrolled in a hospice program cost Medicare $2,737 less than comparable nonusers. For every dollar spent on hospice care, Medicare saved $1.52.

Savings were affected by length of stay in hospice. The greatest savings were for patients served for a 2-month period. Savings decreased for each continuing month of service, but there were still gains at 12 months of hospice care.

Table 1 illustrates adjusted Medicare reimbursement saved per dollar of hospice expenditures. As the median length of stay in U.S. hospices has been reported to be 36 days (Christakis, 1996), it would seem that it would be beneficial for patients to be admitted to hospice sooner than at present. It is also fair to question hospice patients who continue to be in the program for lengthy periods, although there are few of these (<15%).

In spite of the enormous size and scope of the Lewin VH1 study (NHO, 1995a), it has not been taken that seriously by policymakers and industry analysts. Perhaps any study funded by a constituent group has the appearance of being biased toward the proponents' view. Lack of randomization continues to be a concern, as does the overall cost of hospice care and its very comprehensiveness.

Some insurers view hospice as an unnecessary expense. They feel that standard home health agency care is sufficient and that they should not need to pay for such frills as counseling, spiritual support, bereavement follow-up, and education. The prevailing attitude of some managed care proponents seems to be that dying patients and their families ought to just take care of the problem and that the health care system ought not to be that involved. For managed care to save money, there has to be less use of expensive acute care hospitalization.

The idea that home health agencies can take care of any physical problems that must be attended to and the other needs are not important runs into some problems. Home health agencies are trying to do a better job of keeping patients out of the hospital, but their track record is not that good. The average dying patient served by hospice spends only three days in the hospital in his or her last 60 days of life, whereas a nonhospice patient spends 21 days (Illinois State Hospice Association, 1996).

The reason for this difference is most likely that hospices have developed special expertise in handling the problems of terminal illness. Home health agencies in general admit that they are not set up to provide for dying patients. Home health is designed on a rehabilitation model. Intermittent care is provided to help the patient to return to independence. A wound is healed, a diabetic patient is taught to manage medications, or care is provided while a fracture heals. These are the things home health does best.

Home health agencies also care for chronically ill patients. They provide personal care and teaching, treat periods of exacerbation of illness, and try to keep patients out of crisis, but they are trained to use the emergency care system when a problem arises. Home health care staff always contact the physician to report findings when a patient is having a problem. The physician usually cannot solve the problem over the phone without seeing the patient. They are too busy to try to solve the problem themselves, so they routinely have the patient sent to the emergency room for assessment.

Once in the emergency room, the patient undergoes a battery of tests and is brought into the acute care system. Once in this system, there are powerful incentives to continue treatment until the crisis resolves or the patient dies. Often

Table 1

Adjusted Medicare Part A and Part B Reimbursement Saved Per Dollar of Hospice Expenditures, by Length of Enrollment and Month, 1992

	Length of enrollment						
	<1 month	30-59 days	60-89 days	90-119 days	120-149 days	150-179 days	180-209 days
Last Month	1.68	2.46	2.39	2.25	2.34	2.17	1.06
Month 2		1.01	1.35	1.22	1.17	1.16	1.22
Month 3			0.84	0.99	0.91	0.91	0.89
Month 4				0.72	0.83	0.76	0.72
Month 5					0.67	0.70	0.67
Month 6						0.57	0.65
Month 7							0.56
Total for all months after hospice entry	1.68	1.64	1.49	1.29	1.19	1.06	1.03

Note. From: An Analysis of the Cost Savings of the Medicare Hospice Benefit (p.10), by the National Hospice Organization, 1995, Arlington, VA: Author. Copyright 1995 by the National Hospice Organization. Adapted with permission.

the patient's or family's wishes about treatment are ignored or contradicted. If the family insists on trying to limit care, they are sometimes manipulated into continuing the treatment by being made to feel guilty for suggesting a less invasive approach. The catch-22 is that if a person does not want these things done, the person should not have come to the hospital.

All of these dynamics can be avoided by keeping the patient out of the acute care system in the first place. Hospices have learned to manage the crises of terminal illness by appropriate care at home. Orders to manage such crises as shortness of breath, pain, and agitation are obtained in advance. Families are taught about what to expect as the illness progresses. Instead of panicking when a normal part of the dying process occurs, the caregivers feel in control.

Most lay people seek hospitalization because they believe that there are things that can be done in the hospital that cannot be done at home. Hospices show patients and families that there is nothing the hospital can do that cannot be done at home for a dying patient who wants a peaceful demise.

Still more studies are needed to demonstrate that the cost effectiveness of hospice care is not just due to the nature of the people who choose it. Beyond the issue of cost, though, more attention must be paid to the quality and outcome of the care provided. Managed care continues in its zeal to reduce costs, but purchasers of health care are now demanding that satisfaction with services delivered must be high and good outcomes must be achieved.

QUALITY MANAGEMENT

Hospices want to operate effectively. As one of the newest health care providers, they do not have a history of bureaucratic operation. With little outside scrutiny, hospices have been fairly free to be creative in how they function. This has resulted in some very complex operations and some that lack even basic structures. Hospices that are part of a hospital system or a home health agency have tended to adopt the policy, procedure, and protocol systems of their parent organizations. Those that are community based have usually undergone an evolution from very unstructured volunteer-intensive operations to a gradual transition to formal business operations.

In community-based operations, there is a point of transition when the program reaches a certain size. The informal structure begins to fall apart and management is changed. Community-based boards usually hire a nonhospice person with a background in business at this point to introduce the internal structure needed to manage continued growth.

Beyond the basic business tools of having a billing and financial operations department, up-to-date personnel policies, criteria-based job descriptions and evaluation process, management information systems, and so forth, it is helpful to develop a systematic approach to delivering quality care and a continuous approach to improving performance.

Hospice programs still seem to be in the process of transitioning from the older quality assurance (QA) programs to a quality improvement (QI) approach. QA emphasizes structure and process. A lot of effort was focused on ensuring that all the right forms were filled out and in the chart. A lot of data were collected that described the services provided. There was a lot of rechecking to make sure things were done and done according to policy or procedure. The processes of care were examined to see, for instance, whether a care plan was completed with enough individualization to reflect the patient's actual needs.

What was often missing in the QA approach was any look at what was actually happening to the patient or the organization. There was more emphasis on what was wrong without any focus on how to do things right in the first place. As the QI transition occurs, there is an effort to look at the outcomes of care and to design more effective processes. Process redesign techniques have been borrowed from the business world, which has been using total quality management or continuous quality improvement for many years now.

The structure needed for a hospice can be found by using existing standards such as the NHO (1993) *Standards of a Hospice Program of Care* or accreditation guidelines put out by the JCAHO or the Community Healthcare Accreditation Program. There are also additional structures needed for Medicare certification in the United States.

INTERNAL AND EXTERNAL EVALUATION

A hospice can develop its own process for internal evaluation, and this should be done at least annually. A helpful guideline for this can be found in the NHO (1994a) publication *Standards of a Hospice Program of Care: Self Assessment Tool*. For a hospice program to survive in the current health care climate, it is essential that the program continually strive to reinvent itself and to learn from its experiences how to survive and thrive in its environment.

As important as internal growth and change is, it is how a hospice is externally evaluated that determines its success or failure. These are really two sides to the same coin and have to be looked at together. If an external evaluation such as a complaint about care is received, it may trigger closer scrutiny of an internal activity. Ultimately, all external feedback ought to affect internal operations, and vice versa.

One long-standing external evaluation practice involves use of satisfaction surveys. Like many other health care providers, hospices want feedback from those who use their services. A variety of instruments have been developed to measure satisfaction. Most have been directed at the family or primary caregiver and have been sent after the death. These surveys often use a Likert-type 1–5 format with 1 being *very dissatisfied* and 5 being *very satisfied*. Individual hospice programs collect these data and use them in internal evaluation.

The NHO has developed a standardized family satisfaction survey that has been used by several hundred hospice programs throughout the United States.

As expected, the results submitted to NHO indicate a high rate of satisfaction with services. Hospices have reported mean scores for those responding to each question in the 4.5 to 4.8 range (1995–1997).

In most satisfaction research, a leniency bias is found in survey results that tends to inflate scores (Strasser & Davis, 1991). This can be adjusted for as follows: On a 1–5 scale, a provider is doing very well if results are between 4.25 and 4.50. Results between 4.0 and 4.25 are good but not great. Anything below 4.0 should be cause for concern. According to this, results for the hospices that reported data are excellent. Again, there may be some bias in reporting in that those hospices whose results may not have been so excellent might not have sent their data in.

To deal with this variable and to gain more credibility with outside audiences, hospices are moving toward a system of externally collected satisfaction data. In this arrangement, the hospice contracts with an outside firm to collect the data. The family sends the survey to this research firm. The firm analyzes the results and sends feedback to the individual hospice. Results include the individual hospice's report along with a comparison of how they did in comparison to other programs using this service. Such externally collected data are much more convincing to insurers and others interested in knowing how well the hospice is performing.

Family satisfaction after some time has passed is important information and tends to be reliable feedback. Many times, people will not tell their health care providers what they really feel while they are in treatment for fear that it could negatively affect the care they receive (Strasser & Davis, 1991). Unfortunately, if there is a problem it may be a long time before the hospice finds out about it. Hospices also want to know how the ultimate consumer, the patient, feels about the care provided.

A patient satisfaction survey process is being developed through the NHO to obtain concurrent data on patients' experiences in hospice. Some of the methods being tried to elicit useful feedback from patients include asking for forced-choice ratings and forced negative evaluations and outside evaluators who preserve patient confidentiality.

A hospice wanting additional external evaluation can do this a number of ways. It can seek an independent evaluation or it can seek external accreditation from recognized organizations such as JCAHO or the Community Healthcare Accreditation Program. A number of independent consultants are available to evaluate a hospice's operation. These are usually organizational consultants who can evaluate how well a program is operating on the basis of whatever criteria the hospice and the consultant agree on. The quality of the information generated can vary greatly, and hospices should use caution in selecting an external consultant.

To some extent, becoming Medicare certified to provide hospice care is a form of external evaluation. To qualify for certification, the hospice must comply with all regulations pertaining to providing the Medicare Hospice Benefit. The state usually checks the operation annually to make sure all requirements are met. If any are not met, a deficiency exists, and a plan of correction must be developed.

The main form of external evaluation is through accreditation. A hospice voluntarily requests accreditation and is surveyed by staff from the accreditation agency. The survey involves sending a lot of information in advance to the accrediting body. A site visit is arranged, and a number of specialists are sent to visit the program. During the site visit, staff are interviewed, patients are visited, and records and policies are reviewed. At the conclusion of the visit, major findings are presented in a summation conference. The final results of the survey are prepared and sent to the hospice. Any recommendations made by the surveyors are included. A significant recommendation must be addressed for the hospice to be accredited. This is either done through a written response or, if a more serious issue, through a return survey.

Accreditation is becoming an increasingly important issue for hospices. It is the major standard for external evaluation and may be necessary for survival in the future as health care payors and managed care networks look for ways to distinguish between those who ought to be included in a comprehensive care delivery system.

OUTCOMES OF HOSPICE CARE

There is an increasing emphasis on measuring the outcomes of hospice care. There is still a lot of confusion over the definition of an outcome and there are different types of outcomes. One of the best ways of categorizing outcomes comes from the OASIS Project (Center for Health Research, Denver, Colorado), which gives three types: end result, instrumental, and utilization.

An end-result outcome is something experienced by the patient. An instrumental outcome has to do with the effectiveness of the intervention provided or care delivered. A utilization outcome has to do with how much care was accessed or needed. For health care providers, instrumental outcomes are particularly important in that if done most effectively there will be a positive impact on both end results and utilization.

Ultimately, the most important outcome is the end result. An end-result outcome is a change in the health status of the patient over two points in time. Changes in health status can be physiological, functional, cognitive, emotional, or behavioral. They may or may not be related to the care that was delivered.

A health care provider wants to find out if the outcome was related to the interventions delivered. Certain changes are part of the natural course of the illness (i.e., dying patients will usually get weaker as illness progresses). Some risk adjustment may need to be done to control for deterioration and other characteristics.

Hospices try to measure outcomes a number of ways. Most important, they regularly ask the patient to rate how she or he is feeling. Effectiveness of symptom management is critical to the provision of quality care. Because pain or other forms of distress are what the patient says they are, it is only accurate to have the patient do the rating. These ratings are among the best ways to begin to look at the outcomes of the care being delivered.

A 0–10 rating scale is commonly used to measure distress, with 0 being the complete absence of distress and 10 representing the worst imaginable distress. This approach can be used with physical as well as psychological symptoms. In a recent alpha test of multiple ratings taken from multiple patients by 11 hospices, average pain scores in the last 30 days of life while in hospice ranged from .51 to 4.1. The average for all programs was 1.67 (NHO, 1995d).

Attempts to measure psychosocial and spiritual care outcomes have been particularly difficult to do successfully. Simply measuring levels of distress is descriptive, but there are too many variables to understand the information. For example, in one informal study (Connor, 1996b), social workers asked patients and family members to rate their anxiety levels on a scale ranging from 0 to 10. Results showed that families were most anxious and that the levels tended to increase as death neared.

Population data varied widely, and rater differences were difficult to control. Some experienced social workers seemed to get higher distress levels from their families. This may have been due to their ability to get family members to open up more about their feelings and fears rather than measuring their ineffectiveness at managing anxiety.

Such problems are not unique to hospice. The mental health system also has much difficulty in measuring outcomes. Bereavement care poses similar challenges. The principal measurable outcomes for the bereaved are mortality, morbidity, and use of health care resources. Spiritual care may offer an even greater challenge. There are no objective measures of spiritual growth currently in use.

For those intangible aspects of care, some have used the presence or absence of certain self-statements indicating psychosocial or spiritual resolution, absence of interpersonal conflict, or presence of inner peace. Much more work needs to be done on measurement of such internal processes or states. Researchers could also make greater use of qualitative indices rather than always looking for quantitative measures.

Studies such as these begin to give researchers a way to see how well hospices actually do in the task of managing the dying process. Carefully collected data on symptom control will help to show how good hospices are, and this can be compared with data on care provided outside the hospice venue. Also needed are reliable data on a hospice's impact on the quality of life of its patients. Hospices rate measurement of quality of life as their number one research interest (NHO, 1997b).

QUALITY OF LIFE

Quality of life is an elusive construct that has been hard to measure. There is not a universally agreed-on definition for quality of life. Most would agree that quality of life has two fundamental components, multidimensionality and subjectivity (Cella, 1994). It is multidimensional in that it includes a broad range of domains of experience, including

- psychological functioning
- social functioning
- physical functioning
- family well-being
- side effects and symptoms
- sexuality and intimacy
- treatment satisfaction
- transcendent concerns

It is also fundamentally subjective in that it can only be understood from the patient's perspective. Efforts to estimate quality of life by rating overt behavior fail because they neglect the underlying cognitive processes that mediate a person's perception of quality of life. These include perception of the illness, perception of treatment, expectations of self, and cognitive appraisal of the situation.

Quality of life may best be understood as the gap between one's ideal standard for each of the domains of experience and one's actual experience. One's quality of life is higher to the extent that these standards are being met (Calman, 1984). Each patient has a different sense of what quality of life means, and it changes over time and across situations. There has been an explosion of research into quality of life in recent years. Literally hundreds of instruments and measurement strategies have been put forward. In many ways, quality of life has come to be defined by the tools that have been developed to measure it.

Most early attempts to measure quality of life have relied heavily on measuring the patients' functional ability (Karnofsky, 1949; Zubrod et al., 1960). If the patient could perform activities of daily living, it was assumed that there was good quality of life. Research into patients' perceptions of quality of life has revealed that functional ability does not contribute very much to one's sense of quality of life.

Others have devised single-item estimates of subjective well-being or appraisal of quality of life (Bernheim & Buyse, 1984; Gough, Furnival, Schilder, & Grove, 1983). Single-item measures may help give an overall idea of the patient's level, but they lack dimensions and clinical utility.

Some have argued that global quality of life is too large a construct for understanding patients and that researchers need to focus on measuring health-related quality of life (Guyatt, Feeny, & Patrick, 1993; Padilla, 1992). However, if research focuses exclusively on health concerns, it may ignore the dimensions of patients' experience that are most important to their quality of life.

Some suggest that quality-of-life instruments are best if designed for specific diseases (Cella, Lee-Riordan, Siberman, et al., 1990), and some have developed instruments specifically for use in palliative care (Mount & Cohen, 1997). These efforts help to target the issues that are most likely to affect particular patients; however, they must be able to address those dimensions of experience that affect quality of life in all people.

One new approach to measuring quality of life has been developed by Ira Byock in collaboration with the VITAS Healthcare Corporation (Byock & Merriman, in press). The Missoula/VITAS Quality of Life Scale (MVQOL) attempts to measure five dimensions of the patient's experience (symptoms, functional ability, interpersonal relations, well-being, and transcendent). It is a 25-question instrument that can be administered to cognitively intact patients (a 15-question version is also in development).

One of the most important things about the MVQOL is that in answering the initial questions, the patient determines the relative importance of each of these five dimensions of experience to his or her quality of life. This addition makes the MVQOL unique. The remaining questions measure the patient's perception of quality of life in each area and how much it varies from a baseline. The resulting scores can be helpful to clinicians in designing interventions.

If the patient's quality of life is derived from his or her sense of connection with others (interpersonal), then hospice caregivers can help to make sure the patient feels well supported by the extended family. If the patient is focused on the transcendent, it is important to explore the patient's spiritual life and help ensure that any unresolved issues are addressed. Figure 12.1 addresses change in QOL scores for a period of six weeks from the date of admission into a hospice program.

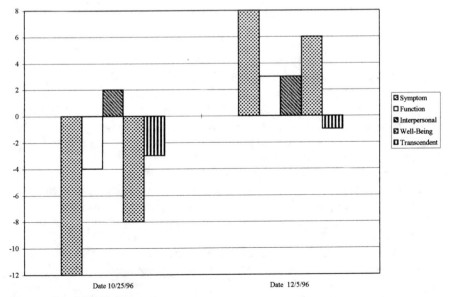

Figure 12.1 MVQOL Dimensions

Quality-of-life tools such as the MVQOL can also be used in measuring care outcomes. If administered on multiple occasions, changes in scores can help the hospice to understand whether its efforts are helping patients to improve their quality of life before dying. Hospices believe that their patients have better quality of life before death but have not been able to demonstrate why, how, or whether this occurs.

Still, the ideal way to measure quality of life in a way that is not too intrusive to the patient, yet gives reliable and valid results, has not been found. Nor has a way been found to account for the significant impact of culture on quality of life.

QUALITY IMPROVEMENT

Hospice programs have been assessing the quality of their services since the hospice movement began. When the Medicare Hospice Benefit was created, it required hospices to assess quality. Efforts to systematically evaluate quality probably began in the United States with the implementation of the JCAHO accreditation program for hospice. Programs were required to implement and document their efforts at QA.

QA standards required the program to measure quality by monitoring important aspects of care. The emphasis was on identifying problems and making changes to programs or operations that would correct the situation. Programs were also required to evaluate their problem-solving interventions to ensure effectiveness.

Individual hospice programs designed monitoring activities and measured their performance at regular intervals. As each program measured quality in its own way, there were no mechanisms to compare results from one program to another. These monitoring results were examined for trends, and programs would strive to improve their performance on the measures chosen.

Medicare and JCAHO suggested certain areas of monitoring such as nursing care and one other discipline or stress management. By and large, it was up to the program to design monitors. The program could measure a structure, a process, or an outcome. JCAHO encouraged programs to work toward outcome measurement, though there was confusion about what an outcome was.

A considerable amount of monitoring activity in hospice was directed at structure and medical records. Programs wanted to ensure that their records were complete and to prove that components of the program were in place. This usually pleased the state surveyors from licensure and certification, although it did little to improve care.

Monitoring in hospice includes looking at important processes and outcomes of care. Many processes are vital to achieving good outcomes. For example, the process for assessing pain is critical to achieve the outcome of pain control. Other monitors used in hospice include, for example, effectiveness in controlling infections; decubitii, or shortness of breath; ability to manage emotional distress; ability to complete advanced directives; accuracy in assessing bereavement risk.

A few years ago, JCAHO began prodding the field to change to the new QI philosophy. They changed their QA requirements to quality assessment and improvement. The emphasis shifted from problem identification to designing systems and processes for quality. The thinking here is why wait for problems to develop, design your care so that problems are eliminated. This comes from the total quality management, continuous quality improvement movement in industry that had so successfully been embraced by the Japanese.

The transition of total quality management from industry to health care has not been smooth. Health care does not exactly run assembly lines, although some patients feel that way at times. Still, the continuous quality improvement emphasis does seem to be an improvement over the old QA system, which did not seem to improve much of what was done. QI is also focused on looking for opportunities for improvement. When a process or aspect of operations seems less than smooth, an improvement group is formed rather than monitoring it to describe what perhaps is already known.

These groups are made up of people who are familiar with the area being studied. The first thing to do is to gain a detailed understanding of the processes involved. The group creates a process map by means of one of a number of tools. After mapping out all the steps and decision points involved, it sometimes becomes apparent how to improve the process. Once the changes are agreed on, the group also has to plan for how to change the process and how to effectively implement the change without creating new problems.

Once the change is carried out, it is necessary to evaluate whether the change has in fact improved the operation. Usually there is an agreed-on measure that will allow comparison of the old method with the new. QI requires good information. In fact, accurate information is the lifeblood of good QI. However, the right information must be collected. Many hospices are coming to realize how limited their information systems are.

The NHO research committee is actively engaged in trying to establish benchmarks for hospice practice throughout the United States. Such a hospice "report card" would include a wide variety of measures on clinical care as well as organizational performance. Some state hospice associations are attempting such benchmarking projects to collect data confidentially from all state providers. Common measures include

- pain control data
- quality-of-life data
- percentage of those dying served in hospice
- demographic data on patients served
- information on location of death
- use of inpatient facilities
- satisfaction with care

- cost per day
- visits per day per full time staff for each discipline
- length of stay data
- ratios that measure visit frequency, bereavement contact, and on-call response

To be effective caregivers, hospices must agree on how to measure the outcomes of care and be able to compare results with those of other providers. They also need to know on an ongoing basis how care is being delivered. It is no longer good enough to look at what happened 6 weeks ago. Hospice needs to know what happened yesterday.

PATHWAYS

A model for treating the whole patient and family is emerging from work done by the NHO's Standards and Accreditation Committee (*A Pathway for Patients and Families Facing Terminal Illness*, NHO, 1997a). In seeking to understand the outcomes of hospice care, this model helps providers understand how hospice care can operate so effectively. This conceptual model attempts to create a common language for providers that can be used to understand and describe the enormous territory hospices deal with in caring for dying patients and their families.

Most pathways in health care have been developed to help improve the efficiency of health care delivery. Health care workers want to get patients in and out of the hospital as quickly as possible with the best outcome. They do not want them to return with the same problem. These pathways are usually centered around particular diseases. If the patient has congestive heart failure, here is how he or she should be treated during a hospitalization or home health stay. Here is how a patient coming into the hospital for a particular orthopedic surgical procedure should be handled.

Hospice care does not fit this model very well. Hospices deal with a variety of diagnoses with different trajectories and no easily determined end point. All have the condition of terminality, so a hospice pathway might best be described as a condition pathway. Each patient and family comes with different resources for coping with the experience and different needs. There is, however, a territory that must be understood for good hospice care to be delivered.

As the patient, the family, and the patient–family unit are assessed, hospice workers need to ensure that they are looking at all the dimensions of the patient's experience. This conceptual framework can help hospices ensure that they are looking at the whole patient–family system.

When hospices intervene, they are either treating, preventing, or promoting. By treating, they are eliminating or lessening a problem by using skilled assessment and therapeutic intervention. By preventing, they avoid a possible problem through skilled assessment or therapeutic intervention. By promoting, they are encouraging growth or a higher level of health through skilled assessment or therapeutic intervention.

Much of hospice work is preventative. Problems do not happen just because of good assessment, prophylactic intervention, and education. This conceptual model helps hospices to understand which areas of the patient's and or family's experience they are dealing with. Dying is more than a medical event, it is also a personal experience. Hospice care is more than medical treatment of pathology. It can also be a time of opportunity and growth. Much of the potential of hospice care is in promotion of health and growth at the end of life.

Using NHO's conceptual grid, hospice achieves the best outcomes through an interdisciplinary assessment of the patient and family states. Each state has associated problems and opportunities associated with it. Patients experience dying in four different states: disease, symptoms, adaptation, and function. Figure 12.2 illustrates the states as experienced by both the patients and their families.

Although hospice does not attempt to cure the patient of his or her disease, it is important for them to understand where the disease is in terms of progression. They also have a responsibility to know when the disease may be improving so that appropriate treatment can be provided. It is also important to understand the effects of secondary diagnoses and comorbid factors that affect a patient's disease state.

The symptom state is the subjective manifestation of the disease state. The kinds of problems or conditions assessed range from sensory or neurological problems to nutritional problems, to fluid balance problems, to elimination problems, to integumentary problems, to cardiac or circulatory problems, to respiratory problems, to immunological problems.

In the adaptive state, hospice focuses on coping, grieving, and existential problems as well as opportunities for growth or higher levels of wellness. The functional state includes a person's physical, cognitive, or social capacity to communicate, learn, and carry out activities of daily living or care requirements. The kinds of issues addressed include physical mobility and compliance.

The family members are not terminally ill, so they do not experience the disease or symptom states. Hospices do need, however, to address their adaptive and functional states. The family's adaptive ability is their ability to emotionally, or spiritually, adjust to the changing environmental conditions or life circumstances. Issues addressed include problems in coping, grieving, and existential concerns as well as opportunities for growth through the experience. The family, too, has different levels of ability to participate functionally. Some may be able to assist in care, and others may not be able to comply with the demands of the situation. Some patients may have no caregiver.

The primary issue for the patient–family unit is their resource state. These are their environment and financial resources related to the provision of patient

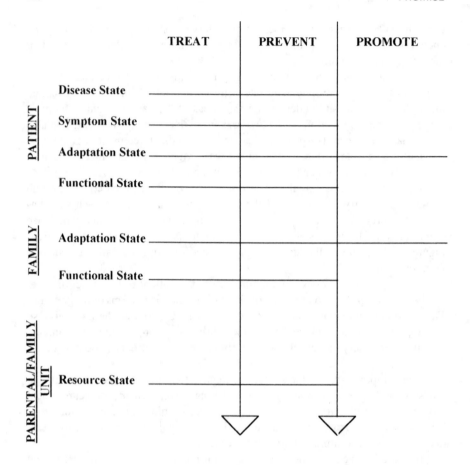

Figure 12.2   Hospice Patient/Family Grid

care and future family health. Issues addressed include safety, shelter, inadequate finances, lack of directives regarding care, unresolved estate, funeral plans, or finances, and legal or custody concerns.

Having a more complete assessment of the patient and family is critical to achieving the primary outcomes for those facing terminal illness. The NHO document (1997a) gives three primary outcomes for the patient and family:

- self-determined life closure
- safe and comfortable dying
- effective grieving

Within these three major areas, many specific measurable outcomes can be found. Ultimately, what hospices are trying to achieve is for persons anticipating their death from a life-threatening illness to remain safe and comfortable until death, supported in life closure as they conceive it by family caregivers, volunteers, and professional staff whose needs for education and counsel are appropriately met.

Whether the hospice movement survives and thrives or becomes a footnote in the history of medicine may be determined by how well it is able to demonstrate the effectiveness of the care it provides.

In the next and final chapter, issues for the future of hospice care are explored.

Chapter 13

The Future of Hospice Care

"The riders in a race do not stop when they reach the goal. There is a little finishing canter before coming to a standstill. There is time to hear the kind voices of friends and to say to oneself, 'the work is done.'"

—Oliver Wendell Holmes, Sr.

There is a fair amount of angst within the hospice community about the future of the movement. Should efforts be focused on becoming more integrated within the health care system, or should hospice remain a separate entity? There is heightened social interest in care at the end of life and a sense that hospice may not be up to the task of changing the way people die in the United States.

Some of this is reflected in the debate over use of the name *hospice*. There are some, both in Europe as well as North America, who would prefer to abandon the term. They feel it has become too self-limiting and that some negative connotations have become associated with it. These negative connotations boil down to *hospice = death*. The self-limiting concerns relate mainly to restrictions on access to hospice brought about by creation of the Hospice Medicare Benefit in the United States and a tendency in other countries for access to hospice to be limited by cultural factors or economic conditions.

In place of *hospice*, the broader term *palliative care* has been suggested. This is put forward to offer the advantage of being a broader frame; you do not have to be dying to get it. It is also more descriptive for what a hospice actually does. The dilemma, however, remains that no matter what it is called, it is still something associated with dying.

The word *hospice* has offered some advantages. It is an ambiguous word. It allows the communicator an opportunity to explain what is meant. It is also a metaphorical term. Death is alluded to indirectly through the comparison of a way station on life's last journey. The name problem is a societal one that simply reflects the continuing lack of ability to integrate the reality of death into our cultural experience.

WHO ARE HOSPICE'S PATIENTS?

Who ought to receive hospice care? When ought they to receive it? What should they receive? These questions have only been partly answered. The broadest frame is that anyone dying ought to have the opportunity of using the services of a hospice.

Dying is a process, not an event. Therefore excluded are people who die unexpectedly in accidents or of undetected illnesses such as a sudden unexpected heart attack. Also excluded are those whose acute conditions have a likely chance of cure. A patient with an acute attack of appendicitis may die, but one would not want to admit the patient to hospice. The whole arena of infectious disease has become more interesting of late.

Many AIDS patients benefit from hospice care, but hospice would not think of admitting a patient with a tropical infectious disease. Hospices may have to rethink how to handle a world where large numbers of people begin dying of new untreatable infectious diseases. It is interesting that once one subtracts all those who, owing to the nature of their situation, are not appropriate for being helped by a hospice, one may be left with a minority of those who die.

A best estimate is that only somewhere around 40% of those who die in a given year are appropriate for hospice care under the current limitations. These are, of course, most of the cancer patients, those dying of other progressively fatal nonmalignant diseases, and many of those dying of progressive chronic illnesses, all of whom would reach a point where they choose not to continue pursuing curative or prolongative treatment.

Of course, this percentage is likely to grow in the years ahead due to advances in the treatment of acute conditions. Before World War II, people tended to die young. Now, society is faced more and more with death from chronic conditions in elderly persons that progress over a long period.

In the United States, hospice currently cares for about 20% of all deaths (NHO, 1996a). In the United Kingdom, hospice cares for about 11% of all deaths. Although there are still large numbers of people who need hospice care and are not getting it, it is also not fair to say that the hospice movement is too small, marginal, or unavailable. At least one third of all cancer and AIDS patients dying in the United States receive hospice care before death.

The defining issue as to who in this group receives hospice care is more and more determined by what sort of treatment they receive. For cancer patients, if the treatment is aimed at curing the disease or achieving a remission, they do not enter hospice. The same is true for most other conditions. If the aim is survival, then hospice is not considered an option. An increasing number of patients are seeking survival, no matter how unlikely the odds, and never getting hospice.

Changing the name to palliative care would not address this issue. If a person is seeking survival, he or she does not just want symptoms managed. The person will settle for no less than cure or at least an uncertain future. Once given the label of being terminally ill, a person's future has been determined; there is no mystery about it—the person is expected to die. Staying in the gray area at least gives the illusion that all options remain open.

This brings us back to a fundamental question about the nature of hospice care. Is it necessary for every patient to acknowledge the fact of their dying to be served by hospice? Can there not be room for some uncertainty and mystery as they face the abyss? This is perhaps where things have gone amiss in hospice's efforts to fit into the health care system and to help patients to face reality. Hospice has become too identified with death rather than life.

It has always been said that hospice is about living, not dying. Yet, U.S. hospices embraced the Hospice Medicare Benefit with its requirement of a 6-month prognosis for admission. This has put hospice in a box with regard to treatment choice. The patient has to choose to stop receiving anything but palliative treatment. This means that the whole spectrum of patients who want to keep some option of survival open have been excluded from hospice. Patients still have a choice, but if they are dying and choose something other than symptom management, they cannot have hospice.

Some in hospice have come to take the Medicare benefit to be the definition of hospice. This puts the cart before the horse. It is not uncommon to hear comments such as "He doesn't belong in hospice" when talking about a patient who wants to continue chemotherapy or "She is not hospice appropriate" when referring to a patient who cannot agree to a DNR order.

People who are intent on cure may not be appropriate for hospice, but there are many who struggle with letting go of hope for survival. They may feel pressure from their family to keep fighting. These people may be more in need of hospice support than those who are seemingly accepting of their terminal condition.

CHILDREN

Most hospices provide care for children. There are even hospices that specialize in the care of children. Some hospices have developed pediatric hospice teams. The care of a dying child requires extraordinary sensitivity and specialized knowledge of palliative care. There has also been a tendency to be more flexible about some of the admission criteria adults are held to. Many children come into hospice while still receiving aggressive treatments. Their need to maintain hope for improvement is better tolerated by hospice workers. Many psychosocial resources are brought to bear, including, in some cases, expressive or art therapy to help the patient or siblings in their expression of grief.

CHRONIC CARE

Health care in the United States is organized to provide primarily acute care services, whereas the greatest need is for chronic care. The system does not effectively meet the needs of those suffering from health care problems. It is estimated that 99 million persons in the United States have chronic conditions, of whom 41 million have limitations owing to their condition.

Only 5.3% of U.S. deaths in 1990 were from infectious diseases; 4.2% were from accidents. Cardiovascular disease was the cause of 42% of deaths, and 23.2% of deaths were from cancer. The remaining 25.3% were from other causes. All together, chronic conditions account for three out of every four deaths (Robert Wood Johnson Foundation, 1996).

More than half (55%) of all emergency room visits are made by people with chronic conditions. Hospital care is predominately being provided to people with chronic conditions: 80% of all hospital days and 69% of all admissions are for chronic care. Virtually all home health care (96%) is given to chronically ill persons. People with chronic illness sometimes receive care that is more intensive, more specialized, and more expensive than they need or want.

ISSUES FOR THE FUTURE OF HOSPICE CARE

Hospices need to be more adaptable in providing services to dying patients that are outside the boundaries of current practice

If the patient does not qualify for a standard hospice benefit, there may be other ways of providing services. Many hospices are experimenting with "prehospice" programs that meet the physical, emotional, or spiritual needs of patients who have a life-threatening illness but may not have a 6-month prognosis. Services should be designed to meet the needs of special populations of patients facing the end of life. Hospices should be careful that the intent of providing these services is to meet a need rather than to provide free services as a way of inducing referrals.

Hospice has a great deal to offer the health care system in the management of terminal and chronic life-threatening illness. There could be a way for the boundary to be expanded so that appropriate services could be provided and reimbursed for hospice to manage a variety of seriously ill patients. For example, hospice could receive a small case management fee to help manage the care of patients with congestive heart disease, dementia, or pulmonary diseases. The fees paid could be considerably less than the current payment for treating these illnesses. Hospices could provide more daycare services.

The patient and family would be educated about home management of care and how to handle crises. Services could be provided during periods of exacerbation of illness. The 24-hours-a-day hospice on-call service would be available, and the aim would be to keep the patient stable at home instead of in the hospital. At the point where the disease progresses to endstage, they could be admitted to the regular hospice service.

In the United Kingdom, an effort is being made to promote three levels of palliative care to broaden the availability of services. The first level is the promotion of a palliative care approach within the general health care system. All practitioners ought to have a general knowledge of palliative principles. The second level is creation of consulting palliative care services that would be available to provide some interdisciplinary services within the health care system. This would be along the model developed at St. Lukes Hospital in New York. A consultation team would be available to see patients having symptom management problems, usually in a hospital setting.

The third level of palliative care would be a specialty interdisciplinary palliative care service. This would be the service that is currently provided by hospice facilities throughout the United Kingdom. It would offer the full range of hospice services on an inpatient basis and would include home visitation as well as day care services.

Hospices need to be more responsive to diverse cultural groups

The hospice movement in the United States continues to serve a predominantly white population. There is a rich diversity in our society of different responses to death and dying. More effort is needed to understand these differences and to develop hospice services that respond to the unique interplay of culture and religion found throughout our society.

Hospices will need a different mix of resources to effectively care for more dying patients and have a greater impact on end-of-life care

Many people are not admitted to or served by hospices because their need for care is more than the hospice can deliver. This includes many patients who live alone, those without primary care providers, and those with complex or devastating complications of illness. Many of these patients remain in the hospital during their last weeks. Hospices need a way to provide around-the-clock care to selected patients to help them die at home. The continuous care provisions under the Hospice Medicare Benefit are too restrictive and are only available for brief periods of severe crisis. What is needed are greater amounts of practical nursing assistance.

To help determine how to best serve patients at various points in the end-of-life continuum, better prognostic tools are needed

Hospices have relied on the judgment of community physicians and their own experiences to make decisions about whom to serve. This has led to a situation in which most patients are admitted far too late for effective treatment and a few are admitted too soon.

Efforts to continue the development and revision of *Medical Guidelines for Determining Prognosis in Selected Non-Cancer Diseases* (NHO, 1996b) should be supported. Additional research on prognosis needs to be funded and conducted. At present, the available prognostic guidelines are based on limited science. They will need continual revision as knowledge is added to the literature. Rather than using a set time frame of 6 months for hospice admission, medical criteria that suggest death in weeks or months rather than years should be used.

Specialization in the field of palliation will help improve acceptance of the developing body of knowledge about care of the dying

Although there is a general trend toward decreased specialization and increased emphasis on primary care in medicine, there is a need for the recognition of palliative care as a unique discipline. This could be accomplished a number of ways, including through the creation of a diploma in palliative medicine or through the recognition of palliative care as a subspecialty.

The Academy of Hospice and Palliative Medicine now offers a certification for physicians. In the future, a diploma in palliative medicine could be offered to any physician wanting to gain a working knowledge of palliative care. Existing models and curriculums for a diploma program are available from Canada and the United Kingdom. It would involve mainly self-study while the physician continues to practice, supplemented by periodic on-campus and practicum learning.

Rather than being considered another limited specialty, palliative medicine ought to be viewed as another area of primary care. There is certainly no shortage of patients whose needs are best addressed through palliative care. Many unneeded specialists could consider changing areas of practice to specialize in palliation.

There is some support developing for the recognition of palliative medicine as a distinct specialty. If this were to occur, training programs could be developed, along with intern and residency programs. Physicians trained as specialists in palliative medicine would be able to assist in hospices as well as provide needed assistance in the acute setting for patients who pose particularly difficult challenges in symptom management.

Beyond the physician training needed, there is a need for palliative care principles to be part of the basic curriculum of all health care disciplines

Hospice and palliative care services are by definition interdisciplinary. Each of the health care disciplines needs to incorporate both experiential and didactic learning for disciplines such as nursing, social work, psychology, chaplaincy, and the various therapies.

The effectiveness of clinical work done in hospice and palliative care must continue to be rigorously assessed

The growing body of literature on care of the dying needs to be greatly expanded. The real outcomes that are important in the care of dying patients have only just begun to be identified. Hospices must understand which outcomes are the most significant in the care of patients and to the health care system. There needs to be widespread agreement on how to measure these outcomes accurately and benchmarks for acceptable care outcomes.

Large-scale collection of accurate data on the effectiveness of hospice care is needed to verify claims for the superiority of services that have to date have been based largely on anecdotes. Although it may be easier to measure the outcomes of physical care, it is also critical that the clinical efficacy of psychosocial and spiritual care be examined. Hospices may believe that their current practices are the best, but this ignores the possibility of even better prevention and management of distress.

Providing emotional support is not enough

In the psychosocial arena, there continues to be a lack of specificity to the interventions used in helping patients with their interpersonal and inner distress. Clinicians need to accurately assess the patients' realms of suffering and respond in ways that are focused on their real needs. Hospices have plans of care, but the psychosocial component is rarely well developed. All team members need to understand the patient's and family's psychosocial and spiritual care needs. Every member of the team should deliver consistent interventions based on a strategy that targets the patient's and family's needs and goals.

If the patient is suffering emotionally because of isolation, the team ought to respond with interventions that bring more human contact into the patient's life. If the patient is anxious about suffocating, team members need to reassure the patient, explain how breathlessness can be managed, and help the patient to learn relaxation and breathing techniques that will reduce symptoms and increase sense of control.

Hospice caregivers need to allow for the possibility that the time around dying can include personal growth and an enhanced sense of well-being for the dying person and family

It is easy to stay too focused on the problems that attend the dying process. After physical symptoms are well managed, some people may be able to continue the human developmental process and use the end of life as a time of resolution, appreciation, and closure. This takes hospice beyond the prevention and treatment of negative outcomes to the promotion of positive outcomes for the people served. This ability to create something good out of adversity is one of the things that distinguishes hospice from other providers.

Hospices need to be more vocal in bringing the palliative care perspective to the societal debate on euthanasia and PAS

Too often this debate is presented as a dichotomy between those who believe death is a fundamental right and those who believe it is a fundamental wrong. Hospice occupies the middle ground in this debate and has been largely ignored. The hospice and palliative care perspective needs to be promoted through aggressive advocacy and education efforts at the grass-roots level as well as on the national stage.

Greater support for hospice and palliative care needs to come through government policy

The lack of support for care of the dying in the United States is a national tragedy. Creation of the Medicare Hospice Benefit has gone a long way toward making hospice care accessible to larger numbers of people. However, the growth of the hospice movement is limited, and the care of most people dying is still poor and sometimes terrible.

The SUPPORT Investigators (1995) study has documented that most terminally ill people in hospitals are still faced with dying in pain while their treatment wishes are ignored. In spite of the people served by hospices, most are still dying in these hospitals or institutions.

With the exception of a small program through the National Institutes of Health to develop training programs in hospice and palliative care, there have been no significant government research resources committed to furthering knowledge of palliative care. Enormous sums are provided for research into the treatment of disease, with little success to date. Meanwhile, hundreds of thousands of people die each year with inadequate management of their conditions. The lack of support for palliative care research in the United States ought to be viewed as a disgrace.

In the United Kingdom, those served by hospices remain a fairly small minority of the dying. The National Health Service provides some support to the hospices, but they remain too dependent on philanthropy to reach the great majority of the dying.

Governments concerned for the welfare of citizens ought to promote policies that encourage the use of hospice care. At present, the U.S. health care system is still in many ways motivated by profit to overtreat dying patients. Home health agencies are penalized if they refer a patient to hospice, private physicians have billing difficulties if the patient is on the hospice benefit, hospices are penalized by the fiscal intermediaries or the inspector general if they admit a patient too soon and the patient outlives his or her prognosis, and nursing homes are encouraged to provide skilled nursing services to their dying patients rather than allowing hospice to deliver the care.

Home health agencies have no incentive to refer patients to hospices when it means less income for them. Hospital discharge planners are too busy to work up a hospice referral. They have to deal with how informed the patient is and what his or her goals for care are. All these limitations combine to inhibit the growth and development of hospice care. There is considerable room for policy changes that will promote the success of the hospice movement.

Hospice care needs to become an integral part of the health care system in each country served

Many of the above problems derive from the difficulties in introducing hospice care into an existing health care system. Each country in the world has unique aspects to its health care delivery system. For hospice care to succeed, it must adapt somewhat to the needs of the existing system. There are few countries where care of the terminally ill is already done well. An assessment of how the existing system cares for people dying will usually reveal many unmet needs for education and caregiving.

HOW DOES HOSPICE FIT IN THE HEALTH CARE SYSTEM?

Hospices developed to redress the reality of insensitive care for dying patients. There was a tendency to reject mainstream medicine and to be perceived as rebels. Although this may have been necessary 20 years ago, it is counterproductive today. Hospice needs to embrace the health care system and work for inclusiveness. One of the reasons its voice is not heard loudly in the debate on end-of-life care is that hospice is not taken seriously by the powers-that-be in health care.

There is a perception that hospice is not relevant or having much of an impact. The original goal of putting hospice out of business is not one that will be realized anytime soon. Maybe in another 20 years, health care will be so well integrated that the values and practices of hospice care will be built into the system. There may always be a need for someone to specialize in caring for the dying. Human avoidance of death continues to be pervasive in our culture.

CONCLUSION

This book has examined the development and current status of the hospice movement in the United States. Hospice began as a revolution against the way the health care system treats those who are dying. It is now a positive force for excellence in the care of those facing life-threatening illnesses. The movement has spread throughout the United States, Europe, parts of Africa and Asia, and is beginning to emerge in the East (Saunders & Kastenbaum, 1997). Hospice care has taken some distinct forms in the different societies it has emerged in, all with the common focus of providing compassionate care directed at relief of physical, psychological, social, and spiritual distress.

In describing current hospice practice, the focus has been on how the best hospice care is being delivered in the United States. It is important that some of these distinct ways of caring for dying patients are described in detail. Many new organizations and individuals are entering the hospice and end-of-life care area without knowledge of the history of the movement or how to provide effective palliative care.

Beyond the technical aspects of symptom management is a philosophy of caring that is more difficult to convey to new caregivers, who are often hired and thrust into important roles with little more than general orientation to policy and procedures. It is hoped that this book will help some of the thousands of new hospice and palliative care workers who are now entering the field.

Also described have been the real problems facing hospices in the current health care system. Until recently, the hospice movement has enjoyed little scrutiny and the halo effect of an industry formed by unselfish, highly principled people and has been above reproach. The growth of the movement has brought with it many of the same problems of greed seen throughout the rest of the health care system.

The future for hospice care ought to be bright. The U.S. population is aging, as the huge post–World War II generation reaches old age. Current care for most dying patients is terrible, with patients dying in pain, in institutions, and with their wishes for treatment ignored. Hospice care offers the most effective system of caring for dying people available today.

Impediments to access to hospice care must be removed. Much greater effort must be made to educate the public about options for care at the end of life.

Hospice care is at an important juncture. Will it remain on the fringes of the health care system or will it become part of a fully integrated cradle-to-grave continuum of care? Hospices themselves have a lot to say about the outcome. If they rise to the challenge of providing expert care that is based on science and the needs and wishes of the people served, they will have a bright future.

References

Agency for Health Care Policy and Research. (1994). *Management of cancer pain* (AHCPR Publication No. 94-0592). Rockville, MD: U.S. Department of Health and Human Services.

Autry, J. (1991). *Love and profit: The art of caring leadership.* New York: William Morrow.

Avis, N. E., Brambilla, D. J., Vass, K., & McKinlay, J. B. (1991). The effect of widowhood on health: A prospective analysis from the Massachusetts Women's Health Study. *Social Science Medicine, 33,* 1063–1070.

Barry, K. L., & Fleming, M. F. (1988). Widowhood: A review of the social and medical implication. *Family Medicine, 20,* 413–417.

Becker, E. (1973). *The denial of death.* New York: Free Press.

Beilin, R. (1981). Social functions of denial and death. *Omega, 12*(1), 25–35.

Beissler, A. R. (1979). Denial and affirmation in illness and health. *American Journal of Psychiatry, 136*(8), 1026–1030.

Bengston, V., Ceullar, J., & Ragan, P. (1977). Stratum contrasts and similarities in attitudes toward death. *Journal of Gerontology, 32*(1), 76–78.

Bernheim, J., & Buyse, M. (1984). The anmnestic comparative self assessment for measuring the subjective quality of life of cancer patients. *Journal of Psychosocial Oncology, 1*(4), 25–38.

Birenbaum, H. G., & Kidder, D. (1992). What does hospice cost? *American Journal of Public Health, 74,* 689–697.

Blakney, R. B. (1955). *The way of life.* New York: Mentor Books.

Bowlby, J. (1980/1981). *Attachment and loss. Vol. 3: Sadness and depression.* London: Hogarth.

Breznitz, S. (1983). The seven kinds of denial. In S. Breznitz (Ed.), *The denial of stress* (pp. 257–280). New York: International Universities Press.

Bruera, E., de Stoutz, N., Velasco-Leiva, A., Schoeiler, T., & Hanson, J. (1993, July 3). Effects of oxygen on dyspnoea in hypoxic terminal-cancer patients. *Lancet, 342*(8862), 13–14.

Buckman, R. (1992). *How to break bad news: A guide for health care professionals.* Toronto, Ontario, Canada: University of Toronto Press.

183

Byock, I. (1997). *Dying well: The prospect for growth at the end of life*. New York: Putnam.

Byock, I., & Merriman, M. (in press). Measuring quality of life for patients with the Missoula-VITAS quality of life index. *Palliative Medicine*.

Calman, K. (1984). Quality of life in cancer patients—an hypothesis. *Journal of Medical Ethics, 10*, 124–127.

Cappon, D. (1978). Attitudes of the aged toward death. *Essence 2*(3), 139–147.

Cassell, E. J. (1982). The nature of suffering and the goals of medicine. *New England Journal of Medicine, 306*, 639–645.

Cella, D. (1994). Quality of life: Concepts and definitions. *Journal of Pain & Symptom Management, 9*(3), 186–192.

Cella, D., Lee-Riordan, D., Siberman, M., et al. (1990). Quality of life in advanced cancer: Three new disease specific measures [abstract 1225]. *Proceedings of the American Society for Clinical Oncology, 4*(5), 216.

Christakis, N. A. (1996). Survival of medicare patients after enrollment in hospice programs. *New England Journal of Medicine, 335*, 172–178.

Clark, D. (1995). *Looking Forward: Looking Back—A Debate*. Lecture at International Work Group on Death, Dying, and Bereavement meeting, Oxford, England.

Connor, S. (1992). Denial in terminal illness: To intervene or not to intervene. *Hospice Journal, 8*(4), 1–15.

Connor, S. (1996a). Hospice, bereavement intervention and use of health care resources by surviving spouses. *HMO Practice, 10*(1), 20–23.

Connor, S. (1996b). [Results of study of patient and caregiver anxiety levels.] Unpublished data, Hospice of Central Kentucky.

Connor, S., & Lattanzi-Licht, M. (1995). Trauma response questionnaire results. *NHO Newsline*, Nov. 1, (5)21, pp. 4–5. Arlington, VA: NHO.

Dansak, D. A., & Cordes, R. S. (1978–1979). Cancer: Denial or suppression. *International Journal of Psychiatry in Medicine, 9*(3–4), 257–262.

DePree, M. (1989). *Leadership is an art*. New York: Dell.

DePree, M. (1992). *Leadership jazz*. New York: Dell.

Detwiler, D. A. (1981). The positive functions of denial. *The Journal of Pediatrics, 99*(3), 401–402.

Devins, G. (1979). Death anxiety and voluntary passive euthanasia: Influences of proximity to death and experiences with death in important other persons. *Journal of Consulting and Clinical Psychology, 47*, 301–309.

Douglas, C. (1992). For all the saints. *British Medical Journal, 304*, 579.

Falek, A., & Britton, S. (1974). Phases in coping: The hypothesis and its implications. *Social Biology, 21*(1), 1–7.

Feifel, H. (Ed.). (1959). *The meaning of death*. City: McGraw Hill.

Foley, K. (1985). Overview of cancer pain and brachial and lumbosacral plexopathy [syllabus from Management of Cancer Pain postgraduate course]. (Available from Memorial Sloan-Kettering Cancer Center, New York).

Freud, A. (1948). *The ego and mechanisms of defense*. London: Hogarth Press & The Institute of Psychoanalysis.

Freud, S. (1917). *Mourning and melancholia*. In J. Strachey (Ed. and Trans.), *The standard edition of the complete psychological works of Sigmund Freud* (Vol. 15). London: Hogarth Press & The Institute of Psychoanalysis. (Original work published)

Freud, S. (1924). *The loss of reality in psychosis and neurosis*. In J. Strachey (Ed. and Trans.), *The standard edition of the complete psychological works of Sigmund Freud* (Vol. 22, p. 184). London: Hogarth Press & The Institute of Psychoanalysis. (Original work published)

Freud, S. (1940). *An outline of psychoanalysis*. In J. Strachey (Ed. and Trans.), *Standard edition of the complete psychological works of Sigmund Freud* (Vol. 23, pp. 140–207). London: Hogarth Press & The Institute of Psychoanalysis. (Original work published)

Fulton, R. (1965). *Death and identity*. Bowie, MD: Charles Press.

Garfield, C. (1978). Elements of psychosocial oncology: Doctor-patient relationships in terminal illness. In C. Garfield (Ed.), *Psychosocial care of the dying patient*. New York: McGraw Hill.

Glaser, B.G., & Strauss, A. L. (1965). *Awareness of dying*. Chicago: Adeline.

Gough, I., Furnival, C., Schilder, L., & Grove, W. (1983). Assessment of the quality of life of patients with advanced cancer. *European Journal of Cancer and Clinical Oncology, 19*, 1161–1165.

Greer, D., Mor, V., Morris, J. N., Sherwood, S., Kidder, D., & Birnbaum, H. (1986). An alternative in terminal care: Results of the National Hospice Study. *Journal of Chronic Diseases, 39*(1), 9–26.

Grossman, S., Sheidler, V. R., Swedeen, K., Mucenski, J., & Piantadosi, S. (1991). Correlation of patient and caregiver ratings of cancer pain. *Journal of Pain and Symptom Management, 6*, 53–57.

Guyatt, G., Feeny, D., & Patrick, D. (1993). Measuring health-related quality of life. *Annals of Internal Medicine, 118*, 622–629.

Haan, N. (1965). Coping and defense mechanisms related to personality inventories. *Journal of Consulting and Clinical Psychology, 29*, 373–378.

Hackett, T. P., & Cassem, N. H. (1970). Psychological reaction to life threatening stress: A study of acute myocardial infarction. In H. S. Abram (Ed.), *Psychological aspects of stress*. Springfield, IL: Charles C Thomas.

Hackett, T. P., & Cassem, N. H. (1974). Development of a quantitative rating scale to assess denial. *Journal of Psychosomatic Research, 18*(2), 93–100.

Hackett, T. P., & Weisman, A. D. (1964). Reactions to the imminence of death. In G. H. Grosser, H. Wechsler, & M. Greenblatt (Eds.), *The threat of impending disaster: Contributions to the psychology of stress* (pp. 300–311). Cambridge, MA: M.I.T. Press.

Hackett, T. P., & Weisman, A. D. (1969). Denial as a factor in patients with heart disease and cancer. *Annals of the New York Academy of Sciences, 164*, 182.

Hendin, H., Rutenfrancs, C., & Zylich. Z. (1997). Physician assisted suicide and euthanasia in the Netherlands: Lessons from the Dutch. *Journal of the American Medical Association*. June 4; 277(21): 1720–1722.

Hinton, J. (1972). *Dying*. Middlesex, England: Pelican Books.

Holland, J. (1989). Clinical course of cancer. In J. Holland & J. Rowland (Eds.), *Handbook of psychooncology* (pp. 75–100). New York: Oxford University Press.

Horowitz, M. (1986). *Stress response syndromes.* New Jersey: Aronson.

Illinois State Hospice Organization (1996). Hospice Medicaid Fact Sheet. (from United State Health Care Finance Administration data). Chicago: ISHO.

International Work Group on Death, Dying, and Bereavement. (1993). A statement of assumptions and principles concerning psychosocial care of dying persons and their families. In *Statements on death, dying and bereavement* (pp. 43–52). Ontario, Canada: International Work Group of the IWG.

Irish, D.P. (1993). *Ethnic variations in dying, death, and grief: Diversity in universality.* Washington, DC: Taylor & Francis.

Jacobs, S., & Leiberman, P. (1987). Bereavement and depression. In O. Cameron (Ed.), *Presentations of depression.* New York: Wiley.

Joint Commission on Accreditation of Hospitals (1984). *Hospice Standards Manual.* Chicago: JCAH.

Joint Commission on Accreditation of Health Care Organizations (1994). *1995 Accreditation Manual for Home Care.* Illinois: JCAHO.

Kalish, R. (1978). A little myth is a dangerous thing: Research in the service of the dying. In C. Garfield (Ed.), *Psychosocial care of the dying patient* (pp. 219–226). New York: McGraw Hill.

Kalish, R., & Reynolds, D. (1977). The role of age in death attitudes. *Death Education, 1*(2), 205–230.

Kane, R., Wales, J., Bernstein, L., Leibowitz, A., & Kaplan, S. (1984). A randomized control trial of hospice care. *Lancet, 1*(8232), 890–894.

Karnofsky, D. A. (1949). The clinical evaluation of chemotherapeutic agents in cancer. In C. M. McCleod (Ed.), *Evaluation of chemotherapeutic agents* (pp. 191–205). New York: Columbia University Press.

Kastenbaum, R. (1974). On death and dying: Should we have mixed feelings about our ambivalence toward the aged? *Journal of Geriatric Psychiatry, 7*(1), 94–107.

Kastenbaum, R., & Aisenberg (1972). *The psychology of death.* New York: Springer.

Kastenbaum R., & Kastenbaum, B. (1989). *Encyclopedia of death.* Phoenix, AZ: Oryx Press.

Kaye, P. (1993) *Notes on symptom control in hospice and palliative care.* Essex, CT: Hospice Education Institute.

Klass, D., Silverman, P., & Nickman, S. (Eds.). (1996). *Continuing bonds: New understandings of grief.* Washington, DC: Taylor & Francis.

Kübler-Ross, E. (1969). *On death and dying.* New York: Macmillan.

Larson, D. (1993). *The helper's journey: Working with people facing grief, loss, and life threatening illness.* Champaign, IL: Research Press.

Lazarus, R. S. (1966). *Psychological stress and the coping process.* New York: McGraw Hill.

Lazarus, R. S. (1985). The trivialization of distress. In J. D. Rosen & L. J. Solomon (Eds), *Preventing health risk behaviors and promoting coping with illness* (Vol. 8). Hanover, NH: University Press of New England.

Lazarus, R. S., & Golden, G. (1981). The function of denial in stress, coping, and aging. In E. McGarraugh & S. Kiesler (Eds.), *Biology, behavior and aging* (pp. 283–307). New York: Academic Press.

Lynn, J., Tino, J., & Harrell, F. (1995). Accurate prognostication of death: Opportunities and challenges for clinicians. *Western Journal of Medicine, 163*, 1–8.

Maslow, A. H. (1967). A theory of metamotivation: The biological rooting of the value life. *Journal of Humanistic Psychology, 7*, 93–127.

Mor, V., Greer, D., & Kastenbaum, R. (1988). *The hospice experiment*. Baltimore: Johns Hopkins University Press.

Mount, B., & Cohen, R. (1997). Validity of the McGill Quality of Life Questionnaire in the palliative care setting: A multi-centre Canadian study demonstrating the importance of the existential domain. *Palliative Medicine*. Jan.; *11*(1): 3–20.

Murphy, D., Burrows, D., Santilli, S., Kemp, A., Tenner, S., Kreling, B., & Teno, J. (1994). Influence of the probablility of survival on patient's preference regarding cardiopulmonary resuscitation. *New England Journal of Medicine, 330*:8, 545–549.

National Hospice Organization. (1992). Poll says hospice leads. *NHO Newsline, 3*(3), 4.

National Hospice Organization. (1993). *Standards of a hospice program of care*. Arlington VA: NHO.

National Hospice Organization. (1994a). *Standards of a hospice program of care: Self assessment tool*. Arlington, VA: NHO.

National Hospice Organization (1994b). *Guidelines for social work in hospice*. Arlington, VA: NHO.

National Hospice Organization. (1995a). *An analysis of the cost savings of the Medicare Hospice Benefit* (Item No. 712901). Arlington, VA: NHO.

National Hospice Organization. (1995b). *Hospice services: Guidelines and definitions*. (Item No. 712893) Arlington, VA: NHO.

National Hospice Organization (1995c). *Medical guidelines for determining prognosis in selected non-cancer diseases, 1ˢᵗ edition*. Arlington, VA: NHO.

National Hospice Organization (1995d). [Results of Pain Control Study.] Unpublished data.

National Hospice Organization. (1996a). *Guide to the nation's hospices*. Arlington, VA: NHO.

National Hospice Organization. (1996b). *Medical guidelines for determining prognosis in selected non-cancer diseases* (2nd ed., Item No. 713008). Arlington, VA: NHO.

National Hospice Organization (1996c). *Results of NHO provider member census*. Arlington, VA: NHO.

National Hospice Organization (1997a). *A pathway for patients and families facing terminal illness*. Arlington, VA: NHO.

National Hospice Organization. (1997b). [Results of survey on research interests of hospices.] Unpublished data.

Osterweis, M., Solomon, F., & Green, M. (Eds.). (1984). *Bereavement: Reactions, consequences, and care*. Washington, DC: National Academy Press.

Padilla, G. (1992). Validity of health related quality of life subscales. *Progress in Cardiovascular Nursing, 7*(2), 13–20.

Pang, W. S. (1994). Dyspnoea in advanced malignancies: A palliative care approach. *Annals of the Academy of Medicine Singapore, 23*(2), 183–185.

Pattison, E. M. (1978). The living-dying process. In C. Garfield (Ed.), *Psychosocial care of the dying patient* (pp. 133–167). New York: McGraw Hill.

Pijnenborg, L., van der Maas, P., van Delden, J., & Looman, C. (1993). Life terminating acts without explicit request of patient. *Lancet, 341*, 1196–1199.

Rando, T. (ed) (1986). *Loss and anticipatory grief*. Lexington, MA: Lexington Books.

Rando, T. (1993). *Treatment of complicated mourning*. Champaign, IL: Research Press.

Robert Wood Johnson Foundation. (1996). *Chronic care in America*. New Jersey: RWJF.

Rosen, E. (1990). *Families facing death: Family dynamics of terminal illness*. Lexington, MA: Lexington Books.

Sanders, C., (1993). Risk factors in bereavement outcome. In Stroebe, M., Stroebe, W., & Hansson, R. O. (eds.) (1993). *Handbook of bereavement: Theory, research, & intervention*. (255–270). New York: Cambridge University Press.

Saunders, C. & Kastenbaum, R. (1997). *Hospice care on the international scene*. New York: Springer.

Sjoback, H. (1973). *The psychoanalytic theory of defensive processes*. New York: Wiley.

Strasser, S., & Davis, R. M. (1991). *Measuring patient satisfaction for improved patient services*. Ann Arbor, MI: Health Administration Press.

Stroebe, M., & Shut, H. (1995, June). *Dual process model of grief*. Lecture at the meeting of the International Work Group on Death, Dying, and Bereavement, Oxford, England.

Stroebe, M., Stroebe, W., & Hansson, R. O. (eds.) (1993). *Handbook of bereavement theory, research, and intervention*. New York: Cambridge University Press.

Stroebe, W., & Stroebe, M. (1987). *Bereavement and health*. New York: Cambridge University Press.

SUPPORT Investigators. (1995). A controlled trial to improve care for seriously ill patients. *JAMA: Journal of the American Medical Association, 274*(20), 1591–1598.

Taylor, S. (1989). *Positive illusions: Creative self deceptions and the healthy mind*. New York: Basic Books.

Teske, K., Dant, R., & Cleeland, C. (1983). Relationships between nurses' observations and self-report of pain. *Pain, 16*, 289–296.

Wass, H. (1977). Views and opinions of elderly persons concerning death. *Educational Gerontology, 2*(1), 15–26.

Weisman, A. D. (1972). *On dying and denying: A psychiatric study of terminality*. New York: Behavioral Publications.

Wolinsky, F. D., & Johnson, R. J. (1992). Widowhood, health status, and use of health services by older adults: A cross sectional and perspective approach. *Journal of Gerontology, 47*, S8–S16.

Worden, W. J. (1991). *Grief counseling and grief therapy: A handbook for the mental health practitioner* (2nd ed.). New York: Springer.

World Health Organization. (1990). *Cancer pain relief and palliative care* (WHO Technical report series 804). Geneva, Switzerland: WHO.

Wortman, C., & Silver, R. C. (1989). The myths of coping with loss. *Journal of Consulting and Clinical Psychology, 57*, 349–357.

Zerwekh, J. (1993). Transcending life: The practical wisdom of nursing hospice experts. *American Journal of Hospice and Palliative Care, 10*(5), 26–31.

Zubrod, C., et al. (1960). Appraisal of methods for the study of chemotherapy of cancer in man: Comparative therapeutic trial of nitrogen mustard and triethylene thiophosoph oramide. *Journal of Chronic Disease, 11*, 7–33.

Appendixes

Appendix 1
DISCUSSION QUESTIONS AND ACTIVITIES BY CHAPTER

CHAPTER 1: So What Is Hospice Anyway?

1. Who is the founder of the modern hospice movement?
2. What is the principal philosophical basis of hospice?
3. List at least three of the characteristics found in all hospices.
4. Give the name of the largest national organization that advocates for hospice care.
5. Give one major psychosocial issue facing a dying person.

Activity: Visit a hospice program in your community.

CHAPTER 2: The Team

1. What is the preferred type of hospice team functioning?
   (a) unidisciplinary
   (b) multidisciplinary
   (c) interdisciplinary
   (d) transdisciplinary
2. Is the administration part of the hospice team?
3. What is the primary function of the home health aide?
4. Volunteers are primarily used in a professional capacity. Yes or No
5. Counseling is provided by a variety of disciplines. Yes or No

Activity: Interview a hospice team member in your community

CHAPTER 3: Symptom Management and Physical Care

1. What are the two major types of pain?
2. Name three other symptoms commonly dealt with in hospice care.
3. The World Health Organization analgesic ladder is divided into what three steps?

4. Pain is what the patient says pain is. True or False
5. Pain medication should be given whenever the patient requests it. True or False
Activity: Interview a hospice patient or family member.

CHAPTER 4: Psychosocial and Spiritual Care

1. Were Elisabeth Kübler-Ross's five stages of dying an accurate description of how people face death?
2. Is it normal for a dying patient to choose not to acknowledge impending death?
3. When told of their terminal illness, do some patients experience relief?
4. Is acceptance the same thing as resignation?
5. When giving bad news, is it important to ask the patients how much they want to know?
Activity: Arrange to have a grief counselor do a death personal awareness exercise with the group.

CHAPTER 5: Grief and Bereavement

1. What is the minimum amount of time a hospice provides bereavement support to a family?
2. Do most hospices provide bereavement support to the community at large?
3. List two examples of pathological or complicated grief.
4. Give two red flags for complicated grief.
5. Has hospice bereavement follow-up been found to help reduce health care use?
Activity: Visit a funeral home or have the group discuss their reactions to the deaths of relatives.

CHAPTER 6: Community Education

1. Are the advanced health care directives of most dying patients honored when they are in the hospital?
2. Are some hospices involved in responding to trauma in the community?
3. Is there an accepted medical specialty for palliative care?
4. Do many hospices run support groups for cancer patients?
5. Give two topics often found in hospice volunteer training.
Activity: Find out if there are any classes on death and dying offered in the community. Volunteer for a local hospice.

CHAPTER 7: The Realities of Hospice Management

1. Name at least 2 of the 11 chapters in the *NHO Standards of a Hospice Program of Care*.
2. How does managed care help a hospice program?
3. How does managed care hurt a hospice program?
4. What is a per diem payment?
5. What is the difference between a palliative and a prolongative treatment?
Activity: Discuss with your group whether you would want to seek aggressive or palliative treatment if you had an advanced cancer.

CHAPTER 8: The Bureaucracy of Dying

1. Name the four levels of care covered under the Hospice Medicare Benefit.
2. Is it difficult for hospices to determine a patient's prognosis?
3. Is hospice care better quality than traditional care?
4. Are all hospices nonprofit corporations?
5. Is there a medical specialty for palliative medicine?

Activity: Visit a local hospital to see where cancer patients are cared for. Ask about the hospital's relationship with any hospices.

CHAPTER 9: Society in Denial

Activity: Discuss with the group how you would want to be told if you had a terminal illness. How would you respond to this news? Would you want to put it out of your mind or would you want to face it?

CHAPTER 10: A Right to Die?

Activity: Discuss the issue of PAS with your group. Explore the arguments in favor of it and those against it. Discuss hospice's role in the assisted-suicide debate.

CHAPTER 11: Why Hospice Is Unique in the Health Care System

Activity: Discuss with the group whether they see the time before death as a time for personal growth and development. Review some of the unique aspects of hospice care such as prevention of distress, deinstitutionalization, and teamwork.

CHAPTER 12: How Good Is Hospice Care?

Activity: Discuss with the group possible outcomes for hospice care, including measures of symptom distress, quality of life, and satisfaction. See if the group can come up with additional outcomes.

CHAPTER 13: The Future of Hospice Care

Activity: Discuss the future of hospice with your group, using the 12 issues for the future of hospice care given in this chapter.

Appendix 2

ORGANIZATIONAL REFERENCES

American Academy of Bereavement
2090 North Kolb Road, Suite 100
Tucson, AZ 85715
   Provides seminars and certification in bereavement facilitation.

American Academy of Hospice and Palliative Medicine
P.O. Box 14288
Gainesville, FL 32604-2288
352-377-8900
   An international physician-member organization dedicated to providing education, research, and support for physicians.

Association for Death Education & Counseling
638 Prospect Avenue
Hartford, CT 06105-4298
203-586-7503
   A membership organization providing education and certification for clinicians who specialize in death, dying, and bereavement.

Candlelighters Childhood Cancer Foundation
1901 Pennsylvania Avenue NW, Suite 1001
Washington, DC 20006
202-659-5136
   Headquarters for local groups that provide education and support for parents.

Center for Death Education & Research
University of Minnesota
1167 Social Science Building
Minneapolis, MN 55455
   An educational resource center on issues related to death and dying.

Centers for Disease Control AIDS Information Hotline
1-800-342-2437
   General information about AIDS, directory of AIDS treatment and support organizations, and advice and support for people with AIDS or HIV.

Center for Loss and Transition
3735 Broken Bow Road
Fort Collins, CO 80526
970-226-6050
   Provides training programs for bereavement professionals and services to the bereaved.

Compassionate Friends
P.O. Box 3696
Oak Brook, IL 60522-3696
708-990-0010
   Headquarters for local chapters that provide support and education for parents and siblings on childhood loss.

Concern for Dying
250 West 57th Street
New York, NY 10107
212-246-6962
   Information center for death-related information. They also provide copies of model durable power of attorney and living will forms.

Cruse Bereavement Care
126 Sheen Road
Richmond, Surrey
TW9 1UR
United Kingdom
011-44-181-940-4818

The Dougy Center
P.O. Box 66461
Portland, OR 97286
503-775-5683
   Support for bereaved children.

Foundation for Thanatology
630 West 168th Street
New York, NY 10032
   An educational organization providing workshops and materials for professionals working with the dying and bereaved.

Hospice Association of America
228 7th Street SE
Washington, DC 20003
202-547-7424
   A membership organization within the National Association for Home Care that advocates for hospice care.

Hospice Education Institute
190 Westbrook Road
Essex, CT 06426
Hospicelink 1-800-331-1620

Hospice Foundation of America
2001 S Street, NW
Suite 300
Washington, DC 20009
    Promotes education on death, dying, and bereavement through publications and teleconferences.

Hospice Nurses Association
Medical Center East, Suite 375
211 North Whitfield Street
Pittsburgh, PA 15206-3031
412-361-2470
    A membership association for nurses working in hospice care. Offers national boards for certification of hospice nurses.

Make Today Count
P.O. Box 222
Osage Beach, MI 65065
314-346-6644
    A national program providing model educational programs for people coping with cancer and other life-threatening illnesses.

National AIDS Hotline
American Social Health Association
P.O. Box 13827
Research Triangle Park, NC 27709
1-800-342-AIDS
    A 24-hour-a-day hotline with recorded information on AIDS and referral capability for medical care and testing.

National Association for Widowed People
P.O. Box 3564
Springfield, IL 62708
    Promotes support groups and resources for widowed people.

National Cancer Institute, Cancer Information Service
1-800-422-6237
    Offers information about conventional and experimental cancer treatment, trials, and protocols and referral to specialized cancer centers.

National Center for Death Education Library
Mount Ida College
777 Dedham Street
Newton Center, MA 02159
    Offers educational materials and resource directory.

National Funeral Directors Association
11121 West Oklahoma Avenue
Milwaukee, WI 53227
414-541-2500
   Helps to educate about all aspects of care of the deceased.

National Hospice Foundation
1901 North Moore Street, Suite 901
Arlington, VA 22209
703-243-5900
   A nonprofit organization advocating for improved care of the dying. Most U.S.
hospices are members. Educational programs and resources are provided.

National Hospice Organization
1901 North Moore Street, Suite 901
Arlington, VA 22209
703-243-5900
   A nonprofit organization advocating for improved care of the dying. Most U.S.
hospices are members. Educational programs and resources are provided.

National Organization for Victim Assistance
717 D Street, NW
Washington, DC 20004
202-232-8560
   An organization that advocates for the rights of victims of crime and disaster and
provides services to local programs.

Parents of Murdered Children
100 East Eighth Street, Room B41
Cincinnati, OH 45202
1-800-327-2499
   A national organization that provides support and educational information for parents
with murdered children.

Project on Death in America
888 Seventh Avenue
29th Floor
New York, NY 10106
212-887-0150
www.soros.org/death.html

Robert Wood Johnson Foundation
P.O. Box 2316
College Road East & Rt. 1
Princeton, NJ 08543-2316
609-452-8701
www.rwjf.org

Survivors of Suicide
Suicide Prevention Center, Inc.
184 Salem Avenue
Dayton, OH 45406
   A national organization providing services to suicidal people and their families.

Widowed Persons Service
American Association of Retired Persons
601 E Street NW
Washington, DC 20049
202-434-2260
   Focus on providing support groups and resources for the newly widowed.

JOURNALS

American Journal of Hospice & Palliative Care
470 Boston Road
Weston, MA 02193

Death Studies
1900 Frost Road, Suite 101
Bristol, PA 19007
215-785-5800

European Journal of Palliative Care
Hayward Medical Communications Ltd
Essex House
Cromwell Park
Chipping Norton
Oxon OX7 5SR, England

Hospice Journal
National Hospice Organization
1901 North Moore Street, Suite 901
Arlington, VA 22209
703-243-5900

Journal of Pain and Symptom Management
Elsevier Science Co.
P.O. Box 882
New York, NY 10159
212-633-3950

Journal of Palliative Care
Center for Bioethics—IRCM
110 Pine Avenue West
Montreal, Quebec, Canada H2W 1R7

OMEGA: The Journal of Death & Dying
Baywood Publishing Co.
26 Austin Avenue, P.O. Box 337
Amityville, NY 11701

Palliative Medicine
Cambridge University Press
110 Midland Avenue
Port Chester, NY 10573

Index